Positive Therapy

Positive psychology emphasises the need to understand the positive side of human experience, as well as understanding and ameliorating psychopathology and distress. *Positive Therapy* explores the relevance of positive psychology to therapy.

Stephen Joseph and P. Alex Linley argue that therapy is not so much about what you do as how you do it, emphasising the influence of the views we hold about human nature on our approach to therapy, and the importance of the relationship between therapist and client over the technique of the therapist. They consider the full range of positive therapies and illustrate the application of the approach in relation to their own work in the field of posttraumatic stress and posttraumatic growth. Finally, they discuss how positive therapy focuses our attention on the social and political context of our work as therapists.

This book is essential reading for all psychotherapists, counsellors, social workers, coaches and psychologists interested in investigating how they engage with clients, and the implications of this engagement for their practice.

Stephen Joseph is Professor of Psychology, Health and Social Care in the Department of Sociology and Social Policy at the University of Nottingham. His research interests are in understanding how people cope with trauma and adversity and more broadly in positive psychology and its applications. He is also a senior practitioner member of the British Psychological Society's Register of Psychologists who specialise in psychotherapy.

P. Alex Linley is a Lecturer in Psychology at the University of Leicester. He is interested in positive psychology and its applications, especially in relation to psychological strengths, and serves as the Director of the Centre for Applied Positive Psychology (CAPP).

We dedicate this book to Martin E. P. Seligman who initiated the positive psychology movement

and

Carl R. Rogers (1902–1987) who founded the person-centred approach

Contents

Preface

Positive psychology is a new movement among psychologists that emphasises the need to understand the positive side of human experience and what makes life worth living, as well as understanding and ameliorating the negative side of psychopathology and distress. In this book, our aim is to explore the relevance of positive psychology to therapy. We are interested in what positive psychology has to offer us in how we think about the ways in which we work therapeutically with people. All professional psychologists, be they clinical psychologists, counselling psychologists, coaching psychologists, health psychologists, or counsellors and psychotherapists, social workers, and other applied health professionals, will find the ideas of positive therapy of interest. This book is written for anyone who offers psychological assistance to others. We have previously written but briefly on the topic of positive therapy, so the invitation to write this book has given us the opportunity to expand on our ideas and to present them more fully. The ideas of this book are our passion; it is our hope that they will become yours, too.

Stephen Joseph
P. Alex Linley
Warwick
August 2005

Acknowledgements

Grateful thanks to Carol Kauffman and Richard Worsley for their encouragement, helpful advice and suggestions. Thanks also to Tom Patterson for his helpful discussions on person-centred theory and positive psychology. Thanks to Joanne Forshaw at Routledge for her enthusiasm for the project and to Claire Lipscomb, Dawn Harris, and Helen Baxter for overseeing the latter stages.

Chapter 1

Introduction: The positive psychology movement

What is positive psychology? What are the implications of positive psychology for psychological practice? What are the implications of positive psychology for therapy? In this chapter, we will answer the first of these questions by describing positive psychology, and elaborating its early history. We will also briefly touch on the second question, considering something of the implications of positive psychology for psychological practice. In the following chapters, we then go on to explore in more detail what positive psychology can tell us about therapy, and begin to delineate what we understand by 'positive therapy'.

A brief history of positive psychology

The advent of 'positive psychology' as we know it today can be traced back to Martin E. P. Seligman's Presidential Address to the American Psychological Association (APA) (Seligman, 1999). Following a moment of epiphany when gardening with his daughter Nikki (Seligman & Csikszentmihalyi, 2000), Seligman realised that psychology had largely neglected the last two of its three pre-World War II missions: curing mental illness, helping all people to lead more productive and fulfilling lives, and identifying and nurturing high talent. The advent of the Veterans Administration (in 1946) and the National Institute of Mental Health (in 1947) had largely rendered psychology a healing discipline based on a disease model and illness ideology (see also Maddux, Snyder, & Lopez, 2004b). When it comes to understanding problems in living, a considerable amount of time and money has been spent over the years documenting the various ways in which people suffer psychologically, as is evidenced by the Diagnostic and Statistical Manual of Mental

Disorders produced by the American Psychiatric Association (1980, 1994, 2000). But, nowhere near the same effort has gone into understanding what makes life worth living, enjoyable, and meaningful. With this realisation, Seligman resolved to use his APA Presidency to initiate a shift in psychology's focus toward a more positive psychology (Seligman, 1999).

This presidential initiative was catalysed through a series of meetings with both junior and senior scholars who would become the leading voices of the new positive psychology movement, and who began to map out what they saw as a positive psychology research agenda. This was followed by the hugely influential January 2000 special issue of the *American Psychologist* on positive psychology (Seligman & Csikszentimihalyi, 2000). This 'special issue on happiness, excellence, and optimal human functioning' included articles on happiness, individual development, subjective well-being, optimism, self-determination theory, adaptive mental mechanisms, emotions and health, wisdom, excellence, creativity, giftedness, and positive youth development, thereby providing a broad vista of topics that were deemed to be covered under the positive psychology umbrella.

From these beginnings, positive psychology has blossomed enormously, and led to the publication of three major handbooks (Linley & Joseph, 2004a; Peterson & Seligman, 2004; Snyder & Lopez, 2002); four introductory texts (Bolt, 2004; Carr, 2003; Compton, 2004; Snyder & Lopez, in press); a number of edited volumes dealing with a variety of positive psychology topics (e.g., Aspinwall & Staudinger, 2003; Cameron, Dutton, & Quinn, 2003; Keyes & Haidt, 2002; Lopez & Snyder, 2003), and more than 15 journal special issues or special sections, together now with a dedicated journal, *The Journal of Positive Psychology* (see Linley, Joseph, Harrington, & Wood, 2006, for a full review). In addition, there is now an annual International Positive Psychology Summit in Washington, DC; biennial conferences organised by the European Network for Positive Psychology; together with a host of conference themes and sections dedicated to positive psychology.

Hence, positive psychology has arisen from auspicious beginnings, but it is also quite clear from even a brief examination of the research literature that positive psychology did not 'begin' in 1997, or 1998, or 1999, or 2000. Research into positive psychology topics has gone on for decades, and might even be traced back to the origins of psychology itself, for example, in William James' writings on 'healthy mindedness' (James, 1902). In broad terms, positive psychology shares a common heritage with parts of humanistic psychology. Shlien, originally writing in 1956, said:

> In the past, mental health has been a 'residual' concept – the absence of disease. We need to do more than describe improvement in terms of say 'anxiety reduction'. We need to say what the person can *do* as health is achieved. As the emphasis on pathology lessens, there have been a few recent efforts toward positive conceptulizations of mental health. Notable among these are Carl Rogers' 'fully Functioning Person', A. Maslow's 'Self-Realizing Persons'.
>
> (Shlien, 2003a, p. 17)

Maslow, a founder of humanistic psychology, also described a 'positive psychology' and called for greater attention to both the positive and negative aspects of human experience:

> The science of psychology has been far more successful on the negative than on the positive side. It has revealed to us much about man's shortcomings, his illness, his sins, but little about his potentialities, his virtues, his achievable aspirations, or his full psychological height. It is as if psychology has voluntarily restricted itself to only half its rightful jurisdiction, and that, the darker, meaner half.
>
> (Maslow, 1954, p. 354)

Initially at least, positive psychology may not have paid sufficient tribute to its lineage from humanistic psychology, and this led to some criticism from the humanistic psychology community (Taylor, 2001). But this situation has begun to change as the common ground between the two disciplines becomes recognised. In our work (e.g., Joseph & Linley, 2004, 2005a), we have tried to show how positive psychology can learn much from the earlier theory, research and practice of humanistic psychology, and we are encouraged that there is now a growing recognition of how the positive psychology research also provides new empirical support for earlier humanistic ideas (Patterson & Joseph, in press; Sheldon & Kasser, 2001). As we will go on to show, our view is that when positive psychology is applied to therapy, there is much that can be learned from the person-centred theory of Carl Rogers. By combining Rogers' theoretical ideas with more recent positive psychological research, we are able to construct a powerful case that speaks to how we might best work with people in seeking to alleviate their distress and facilitate their fulfilment (see also Joseph & Worsley, 2005a). This is how we understand the role and remit of positive therapy, and it is what we go on to explore in much more detail throughout the book. Before we do so, however, we think it would be useful to answer the question 'what is positive psychology?'

What is positive psychology?

In asking this question, we can think about the following definitions of positive psychology, all taken from authoritative sources on positive psychology:

> The field of positive psychology at the subjective level is about valued subjective experiences: well-being, contentment, and satisfaction (in the past); hope and optimism (for the future); and flow and happiness (in the present). At the individual level, it is about positive individual traits: the capacity for love and vocation, courage, interpersonal skill, aesthetic sensibility, perseverance, forgiveness, originality, future mindedness, spirituality, high talent, and wisdom. At the group level, it is about the civic virtues and the institutions that move individuals toward better citizenship: responsibility, nurturance, altruism, civility, moderation, tolerance, and work ethic.
>
> (Seligman & Csikszentmihalyi, 2000, p. 5)

> What is positive psychology? It is nothing more than the scientific study of ordinary human strengths and virtues. Positive psychology revisits 'the average person', with an interest in finding out what works, what is right, and what is improving.
>
> (Sheldon & King, 2001, p. 216)

> Positive psychology is the study of the conditions and processes that contribute to the flourishing or optimal functioning of people, groups, and institutions.
>
> (Gable & Haidt, 2005, p. 104)

There are certainly core themes and consistencies in these definitions, all emphasise the study of positive experiences. But there are also differences in emphasis and interpretation. The definitions could be misunderstood as suggesting that positive psychology is only about positive experiences. Certainly, there is the recognition that we need more understanding of the positive, but not at the expense of the negative.

> The aim of positive psychology is to begin to catalyze a change in the focus of psychology from preoccupation only with repairing the worst things in life to also building positive qualities.
>
> (Seligman & Csikszentmihalyi, 2000, p. 5)

Hence, a positive psychological perspective on the discipline of psychology is that the focus of scientific research and interest should be on understanding the entire breadth of human experience, from loss, suffering, illness, and distress through connection, fulfilment, health, and well-being. This is especially relevant for therapeutic contexts, since as positive psychologists, we would argue that the role of the therapist is not simply to alleviate distress and leave the person free of symptomatology, but also to facilitate well-being and fulfilment, which not only is a worthwhile goal in its own right but which would then also serve a preventive function as buffers against future psychopathology and even recovery from illness (e.g., Fredrickson, 1998, 2001; Fredrickson & Levenson, 1998).

Thus, a common misunderstanding – and unjustified criticism – has been that positive psychology emphasises the 'positive' at the expense of the 'negative' (Held, 2002; Lazarus, 2003). While this may have been an easy juxtaposition to make (especially given the value connotations of 'positive' psychology), we do not believe it is merited. Indeed, in our own work, we have taken great efforts to emphasise this integration of the positive and negative within positive psychology (e.g., Joseph & Worsley, 2005a; Linley & Joseph, 2003, 2004b). It is important to understand that the aim of positive psychology is to promote a more holistic approach to psychology, concerned equally with both positive and negative experiences, so that ultimately, if successful, the term positive might simply fall away leaving the entire disciple of psychology transformed. There is a need therefore to show how positive psychological approaches can speak not only to fulfilment and happiness but also to trauma and suffering (e.g., Harvey, 2001; Joseph & Linley, 2005b; Linley, 2003; Tedeschi & Calhoun, 2004) and existential issues (Bretherton & Ørner, 2004), thus answering criticisms of Pollyanna theorising (e.g., Lazarus, 2003). Indeed, this is something that we go on to consider in much more detail in Chapter 7.

Applied positive psychology

A major area of future potential for positive psychology lies in its applications, and attention is now being focused on where and how positive psychology may be applied (e.g., Linley & Joseph, 2004a; Peterson & Seligman, 2004, ch. 28; Seligman, Steen, Park, & Peterson, 2005). Elsewhere, we have defined applied positive psychology as the 'application of positive psychology research to the facilitation of optimal functioning' (Linley & Joseph, 2004b, p. 4), and considered some of the problems, issues, and opportunities presented by the applications of positive psychology (Linley & Joseph, 2003, 2004c).

In our view, one of the key developments that positive psychology has brought about is a reframing of the questions in which practitioners may be interested. The role of the practitioner, from a positive psychological perspective, is not only about how to alleviate distress, treat illness, and repair weakness, but also how to facilitate well-being, promote health, and build strengths. Consider, for example, the questions of happiness as a public policy aim (Veenhoven, 2004); the benefit of national indicators of subjective well-being (Diener & Seligman, 2004; Pavot & Diener, 2004); the need to understand the optimal experiences of disabled people, rather than simply seeing them as 'disabled' (Delle Fave & Massimini, 2004); working with offenders in ways that recognise their needs and aspirations, thereby significantly reducing recidivism (Ward & Mann, 2004); the need to balance individuality and community in order to achieve good lives for all (Myers, 2004); and the opportunity of being able to prevent disorder and promote well-being through population-based approaches (Huppert, 2004), much as health psychologists do now with their population-based approaches to obesity and smoking. These initiatives would make for a very different society to the one in which we might live today, and they are united by their positive psychological approach to the issues that are of concern.

These questions pose a much bigger agenda than practitioners have traditionally faced, and raise some profound questions. What is our value position, and who has decided on that value position? Is it one we have freely chosen ourselves, or have we accepted it by default as 'the way things are', or has this value position been forced on us by some external agent? What is our remit as practitioners, and who decides that remit? If, as practitioners, we are employed by organisations, it is they who decide the remit. And in doing so, one can well imagine how the organisation may only choose to invest resource in repairing deficits, rather than building assets. The organisation may not see the relevance of life satisfaction, well-being, or strengths to their work, and be asking the question 'What has this got to do with me?'

From traditional practitioner perspectives, the answer may well be 'Not much, if anything.' But if one adopts a positive psychological perspective, and the shift is towards optimal health rather than just the absence of illness, towards prevention and buffering, rather than treatment and vulnerability, then the focus of 'what matters' shifts considerably. Organisations are likely to only change slowly, but we envisage two routes through which this change may come about. First, it may be 'top down', with enlightened leaders offering a new and compelling vision of what the future may look like, and the changes that this ensues. Second, it may be 'bottom up', with a groundswell of opinion as the outlook and aspirations of the practitioners change and evolve, thereby driving a change in the agenda of their organisations. This second option will take time, and no doubt will be influenced by the training of practitioners, and the outlooks that they develop as a result of their training experiences. As the positive psychology movement takes root more widely and continues to flourish, it is our hope that these changes will evolve such that the positive psychology movement will disappear, because it is simply no longer needed. All psychologists will be positive psychologists. If successful, the aims and aspirations of the positive psychology movement will permeate the research and practice of all psychologists, thereby broadening their focus to incorporate the full range of human experience and functioning, from distress and disorder to well-being and fulfilment.

The plan for this book

In Chapter 2, we will describe what we see as a fundamental assumption of positive psychology. The positive psychology movement has provided the impetus for us to reexamine the fundamental assumptions that underlie the professional practice of psychology. Basically, our assumptions about human nature can be broadly grouped into one of two camps. Either we hold that people are intrinsically motivated by destructive impulses, or we hold that people are intrinsically motivated by constructive impulses. We are referring to deep-seated beliefs that we may not always be fully aware of. Imagine two therapists, both listening to their clients talk about themselves and what has gone wrong for them in their lives. On the surface, it may well look as if they are doing the same thing. But when we look closer this similarity is only superficial. One therapist is listening to their client with the deep-seated assumption that people are intrinsically destructive and that their nature must somehow be controlled. The other is listening with the deep-seated assumption that people are intrinsically constructive and that somehow their nature must be facilitated and given freedom of expression. How a therapist understands what the person in front of them is saying is inevitably coloured by their deep-seated assumptions. Of course, to say that these assumptions can be broadly grouped into one of two camps is to simplify and polarise for the purpose of our discussion what can be much more complex shades of grey.

In Chapter 3, we will discuss what we see as the implication of these fundamental assumptions for therapy practice. It is not our intention to advocate new ways of working therapeutically, but rather to ask what it is to work therapeutically within a positive psychology framework. Here we turn to the person-centred theory of Carl Rogers and explore his ideas as one avenue for the development of a genuinely positive psychological approach to counselling and psychotherapy.

In Chapter 4, we ask whether some therapies can be considered positive therapies. Our answer to this is yes. In particular, those therapies based on the theoretical premise of an organismic valuing process and an actualising tendency appear to be most consistent with what the positive psychology research is now telling us. Here we describe the client-centred school of therapy. Seen through the lens of modern positive psychology, we can see that client-centred therapy as originated by Carl Rogers offers a revolutionary and radical way of working with people. The research evidence has become overwhelming that the self-determination of the client is important, and that it is the relationship between the therapist and the client, not the technique of the therapist, which is important.

In Chapter 5, we consider the range of positive therapies and which of the existing therapeutic practices that might be considered genuinely positive. We recognise that our assumptions about human nature provide a broad platform for a range of therapies, and we discuss those that we think are broadly consistent with the concept of the organismic valuing process, or which offer techniques that the more process-directed therapist might find useful.

In Chapter 6, we discuss the implications of our positive therapy approach for understanding psychopathology. Our approach is a genuinely positive psychological one because it speaks to both the negative side of human experience as well as the positive side. We describe how the meta-theory we are offering rejects the medical model. The implications include the rejection of the medical model of psychological disorders, and in its place the adoption of a model based on person-centred personality theory, with the result that we begin to understand well-being as a continuum. In person-centred theory, well-being is proposed to be a function of the extent of congruence between a person's intrinsic tendency toward actualisation and their self-actualisation, with higher levels of congruence leading to increasing well-being, and incongruence leading to psychopathology. Thus, the model recognises that all people fall somewhere on a continuum from psychopathology to fulfilment. Further, we demonstrate how the adoption of the actualising tendency as a meta-theory for understanding psychopathology and well-being raises questions and challenges that the medical model is not equipped to answer.

In Chapter 7, we discuss our own work in the field of posttraumatic stress and posttraumatic growth to illustrate the positive therapy approach. We describe the organismic valuing theory of growth through adversity, which explains how positive adaptation to threatening events leads to the well-recognised processes of intrusion and avoidance that are found within posttraumatic stress. We then show that the 'completion principle' that is commonly described within theories of posttraumatic stress can be understood as part of the broader actualising tendency, and that following this actualising tendency leads to increases in psychological well-being, and movement towards growth and being more fully functioning.

Finally, we will discuss how positive therapy focuses our attention on the social and political context of our work as therapists. Put simply, we have a choice as professional psychologists to be facilitators of personal growth or to be promoters of social adjustment. Sometimes, personal growth and social adjustment are in alignment and there is no conflict, but in our view more often there is conflict, and as therapists we have a choice to make. Are we to foster personal growth or are we to foster social adjustment? Positive therapy as we envision it is ultimately always about personal growth first and foremost. In our view, many of the problems of living encountered in modern society come about as a result of social forces and the demands of living in materialistic cultures. As a result, it in not always in the interests of our clients to direct them towards better social adjustment. Consider the following illustrative example:

One client, John, a man in his early forties, came into therapy seeking help with his self-confidence at work, saying that his lack of confidence, for example, when it came to speaking up in meetings, was holding him back in his career. During therapy, he also began to discuss what he disliked about his job, and came to the realisation that although he had a potentially rewarding career ahead of him financially, it was not a career that gave him a sense of purpose or joy in his life. He simply did not enjoy his work. It was a career he had fallen into after leaving university. At university he had studied management and accountancy, subjects that had not really interested him but which he had chosen following the advice of his parents. He had always wanted to write, and would have liked to study writing or literature at university, and wondered what his life would have been like if he had chosen this path instead. Over time, John began to develop his self-confidence, but also he became more interested in exploring these other issues, and he began to turn his attention to using his skills in this new direction, enrolling in an evening class on writing, and beginning to work on his writing ideas, submitting one of his stories to a competition.

As this example demonstrates, the positive therapeutic approach we advocate here rests on the idea that the agenda for change comes from the client rather than from the therapist. John's agenda was initially focused on developing his self-confidence in order to progress his career, but over time in therapy he introduced other issues, to do with his earlier choices in life, and with his aspirations to be a writer. The therapist's agenda was to stay with John's frame of reference and to explore those issues raised by John himself. In private practice this was not an issue for the therapist, and it was seen as a mark of success by John that he had begun to 'find himself'.

However, psychologists in employment are often faced with a conflict between the agenda of their client and the agenda of their employer. Working for an employee assistance programme, for example, the therapist may feel under pressure to help the client deal more effectively with issues at work even if these are not the issues most pertinent to the client. Under such pressure, the therapists might inadvertently direct John away from 'finding himself' and keep him 'on track' to dealing with his career issues.

Similarly, and perhaps more obviously, in the British National Health Service (NHS), psychologists are under a great deal of pressure to effectively manage their caseloads in such a way as to satisfy senior management, even if this is not always in what would ideally be the best interests of their clients. For example, there is often pressure for therapists to keep the number of sessions to a minimum, because of the pressures of long patient waiting lists and government targets. This pressure can lead therapists to think of therapy as being successful when the client's social and occupational functioning is no longer causing distress or inconvenience to themselves or to others, rather than when they are truly equipped to flourish in the world. Thus, someone can leave NHS treatment more able to function in the world but still deeply unhappy and troubled by life. In NHS terms, success is helping people to better manage and alleviate their symptoms of distress and disorder. It simply is not the goal of therapists in the NHS to engender happiness and fulfilment. Indeed, more critical voices might say that NHS clinical psychologists serve to maintain the status quo of a dysfunctional society that does not value people, except insofar as they are able to contribute to the workforce of a society driven by materialistic aspirations.

We think that professional psychologists too often sweep these conflicts of interest under the carpet, either allowing them to go unrecognised, or conveniently ignoring them. Our view is that the professions of psychology, counselling and psychotherapy should not simply be agents of social control, but agents of personal growth and social change, and that positive psychology provides a challenge to us all to rethink our positions in relation to these issues. Positive psychology is implicitly political because it asks the question of how we create a healthier, happier, and more fulfilled world for people.

Our personal perspective

Of course, for many, what we have to say is old news: existential and humanistic psychologists, counsellors and psychotherapists, as well as critical psychologists, will have heard arguments like this many times before (e.g., Proctor, 2005; Sanders, 2005). We hope that positive psychology will provide a new vehicle for these voices, so that together we can reinvigorate the discipline of psychology as a whole.

We too want positive psychology to become the mainstream approach to psychology, where all psychologists embrace these new ideas and begin to question the assumptions and values behind what it is they do. Given the approach we take and the importance we place on making personal values explicit – as we understand it, the practice of psychological science is never value neutral – we wish to say a little about our backgrounds and how we came to be interested in positive psychology and this field of enquiry.

Stephen Joseph is a chartered health psychologist, and senior practitioner in the British Psychological Society's register of psychologists who specialise in psychotherapy. Stephen is interested in the application of positive psychology to health and social issues. Alex Linley is an applied positive psychologist with interests in psychological strengths and coaching. Both of us are also academics by profession, involved in teaching, research, and consultancy. We believe that the person-centred personality theory of Carl Rogers offers a holistic paradigm that is integrative of both the negative and positive aspects of human experience, which is consistent with the ambitions of the new positive psychology movement. There is considerable overlap in our interests and approach to working with people, but there are differences too – which we will explore throughout this book.

We do not think that there is one positive therapy, but rather positive therapy refers to a constellation of approaches that all share common principles, most notably that the client is their own best expert and has within them resources for personal development and growth. Both of us share this assumption, and person-centred personality theory is the foundation of our approach.

We also realise that the term person centred is often misunderstood by many psychologists, particularly in the United States, who have not recognised the lasting legacy of this approach, and who think it is a superficial approach of little lasting value. They may lose interest by hearing that we have based our work on this approach. We would emphasise, however, that we could have written this book without mentioning Carl Rogers and the person-centred approach at all – because, as we shall show, there is other substantial theory and research that supports our views. These same people might then be interested, but the story of positive psychology begins with humanistic psychology.

So, both of us adopt person-centred personality theory as the foundation of our approach, but we begin to differ when it comes to practice. We recognise that a variety of ways of working as a psychology practitioner can coexist under the positive therapy umbrella. Stephen, as a psychotherapist, tends towards the more classical approach to client-centred therapy, in which it is the relationship between therapist and client that is seen to be of central importance, whereas Alex, as a coach, is more interested in integrative approaches that draw on other aspects of psychology and psychotherapy, and the use of assessment and intervention techniques.

Thus, our theoretical approach to positive therapy is grounded very much in person-centred personality theory, but we recognise a diversity of approaches in practice. We think the practice of positive therapy can range from the more classical approach to client-centred therapy, through other existential and experiential approaches, to ways of working that make use of cognitive-behavioural techniques and more recent innovations in applied positive psychology and coaching. As we shall go on to argue, it is not *what* you do but the way in which you do it.

What is important is that the task of the therapist is to facilitate this process while maintaining a principled stance of respect for the client's own self-direction and self-determination (Grant, 2004; Levitt, 2005a). We define positive therapies as those approaches that share this fundamental assumption, i.e., that clients have the solutions to their problems within themselves, and when they are able to more fully listen to their inner voice, they will be able to find ways forward in life and toward greater well-being. This is not a new idea, but it is one that we think has been marginalised and misunderstood by mainstream psychology. All the therapeutic approaches we describe offer ways of working that can be employed within this meta-theoretical framework.

Thus, we recognise that we have been here before. The general principles of positive psychology that we ought to apply in relation to human potential, fulfilment, growth, development, and so on, are not new. These topics are at the core of humanistic psychology, although the relationship between humanistic psychology and positive psychology has sometimes been a contentious one (see Greening, 2001; Taylor, 2001). Humanistic psychology is a broad church and there are parts of it we would not recognise as positive psychology, but in our view the ideas of the main humanistic psychology writers, such as Carl Rogers, deserve to be set centre stage within positive psychology (see Joseph & Worsley, 2005a; Sheldon & Kasser, 2001).

In this book, we aim to present an integrative approach to therapy that builds bridges between the earlier ideas of humanistic psychology, and the new and exciting movement of positive psychology.

Chapter 2

Positive psychology, fundamental assumptions, and values

> It is not possible to live as a human being without having an idea of what it is to be human.
>
> (Heelas & Lock, 1981, p. 3)

We will argue in this chapter that our ideas about human nature are at the core of how we practise as therapists. Positive therapy is not so much about what you do, as it is about how you do it. We want to discuss how the positive psychology movement has led us to raise questions about our profession's fundamental assumptions concerning human nature. Positive psychology has shown how much of mainstream psychology rests on a fundamental assumption that human nature is essentially destructive. We look back at the ideas of earlier theorists such as Karen Horney and Carl Rogers and how they proposed more constructive views of human nature that are more congruent with the ideas now emerging from positive psychology.

As we have seen in Chapter 1, in recent years Western psychologists have begun to turn their attention to positive human functioning and the question of how psychologists can help people achieve a more optimal level of health and well-being (e.g., Linley & Joseph, 2004a; Seligman & Csikszentmihalyi, 2000; Snyder & Lopez, 2002). What we will go on to show is that positive therapy approaches aim to help people live to the full, no matter where they are along the spectrum of functioning, from illness and disorder to health and well-being. This new positive psychology contrasts very much with the more traditional emphasis by psychologists on illness and psychopathology. There have always been some psychologists interested in positive human functioning, but most professional psychologists have traditionally earned their living by helping people cope better with their problems rather than helping people to live their life to the full. Psychologists are well versed in the treatment of various so-called disorders and how to help people reduce their levels of distress and dysfunction. Our positive therapy approach aims to revolutionise how professional psychologists think about what they are doing, so that their work is not only about the alleviation of distress and dysfunction, but also about the promotion of well-being and optimal functioning.

As therapists, we have many choices as to how to respond to what a person tells us. We can give advice, ask questions, make diagnoses, reassure, listen, administer tests, or interpret, to name but a few of the ways we might respond in our endeavour to assist the person to make changes in their life. A new client arrives and sits down in the chair opposite us. What do we do next? Jaqui tells us about a humiliating experience at work and bursts into laughter as she recounts the story. Another client, Frances, tells us about abusive experiences in childhood in a cold and matter of fact way. Yet another client, Jennifer, tells us with tears streaming from her eyes how unhappy and trapped she feels in her marriage. How ought we to respond to each of these clients? Should we laugh with our client if we also find their story funny? Should we let our client know how we hear them being so 'matter of fact' in spite of what were clearly very emotionally distressing experiences? Should we let our client know how sad we feel to hear her story?

As we shall go on to show, how we decide how we ought to respond to our clients is a choice that we make, and this choice is based on our beliefs and fundamental assumptions as therapists about human nature and the role of therapy. The first of these is our beliefs around whether, as therapists, we are scientists or artists. Psychologists have traditionally adopted the scientific approach and attempted to deliver therapeutic interventions that, just like any other medical intervention, have been shown to be effective. But in recent years it has also become understood that therapy is not just like taking a pill, it is also the meeting of two people and the relationship that forms between them cannot be ignored. We should not ignore science, but to understand therapy we must know that science is not the complete picture, but that therapy is also an art – an expression of our ability to relate with another person at the deepest levels, to be fully human, and to be able to confront the existential truths that face us all.

Therapy as both art and science

We want to be clear that psychology is a scientific discipline and that the positive psychology movement adopts the scientific method. Our views about therapy have developed out of our understanding of the scientific research evidence. What the evidence tells us, time and again, is about the importance of the relationship between therapist and client (see Bozarth & Motomasa, 2005; Wampold, 2001). However, it is also our view that when we are face to face with another person the application of that research evidence involves artistry, it just is not possible to 'do a human relationship'.

Thus, scientific findings can tell us about the associations between various cognitive and emotional factors, between therapeutic interventions and psychological outcomes, but scientific results are not able to tell us how we ought to interact with other people in the application of that science. Similarly, Brodley (2005a) has argued that psychotherapy is limited as a scientific activity because whether we are conscious of it or not, psychotherapy is always an expression of our values and attitudes. Certainly we think therapy must be informed by scientific research, but in our view the practice of therapy is an art. As Wampold (2001) put it so well:

> The performer's grounding in music theory is invisible to the audience unless the canons of composition are violated in such a way as the performance is discordant. Similarly, the master therapist, informed by psychological knowledge and theory and guided by experience, produces an artistry that assists clients to move ahead in their lives with meaning and health.
> (Wampold, 2001, p. 225)

Fundamental assumptions

It is important to understand the process of therapy intellectually, but that in itself does not make for effective practice. Similarly, it is important to have people skills, but that too, in and of itself, does not make for effective practice as a therapist. Artistry arises through the skilful application of theory. What we will now go on to argue is that how we decide on our artistry depends not so much on facts and figures, but ultimately on our fundamental theoretical assumptions about human nature.

This is not a novel idea, since all experienced therapists understand that there are different therapeutic schools, all of which are founded on basic assumptions about human nature (see Joseph, 2001, for a review of the therapeutic models). However, we would argue that mainstream professional psychology approaches have become so entrenched in the use of cognitive-behavioural techniques within the medical model, to the exclusion of other therapeutic approaches, that it is easy to lose sight of the fact that what one does is founded on basic and very deep seated assumptions about human nature.

Each of us has deep-seated beliefs about human nature. For example, some people believe that God created us all and that human nature is divine whereas others believe that we are the products of evolutionary forces and human nature is instinctual. Whatever the truth is on this issue, the fact is that different people believe different things, and what people believe has a profound influence on how they choose to live their lives (see Box 2.1).

Box 2.1 Exploring your assumptions about human nature

Here are some statements about human nature. Read each one and respond quickly as to whether you think it is true or false. Don't think too hard about your answer, give your instant reaction, just respond as quickly as you can, and let your heart say yes or no to each of the following statements.

> People are basically generous
> People are basically selfish
> People are basically greedy
> People are basically kind
> People are basically loving
> People are basically bad

The immediate reaction of some people on reading these statements is true, false, false, true, true, false. For other people, their gut reaction is false, true, true, false, false, true. Other people have a more mixed response, but essentially people fall into one of two categories on reading these statements: either they have what might be characterised as a *positive* view of human nature, or they have what might be characterised as a *negative* view of human nature. Your gut reaction to these statements will possibly tell you something about your own philosophy of human nature, whether you have a basically negative or positive view of human nature.

Few people will not have stopped at some point to think about human nature, and to ask themselves whether people are basically selfish and greedy or whether people are kind and generous. But what is important is to understand just how deep seated and influential your beliefs are. Even if a person has never consciously stopped and asked themselves these sorts of question, deep within themselves they have decided their answer. Why this is important is because each of us lives our life as if what we believe is true. We all have our own way of looking at the world, and while we are looking through our own eyes, it can be hard to imagine that the world could be any different to how we see it. The fact of the matter is that there are many conflicting views on human nature, with many religious leaders, scientists, philosophers and psychologists all holding different views on human nature. Our beliefs about human nature are so deep seated that we rarely question them, and yet they fundamentally influence our attitude towards people and our understandings of why people do the things that they do. As therapists, our fundamental assumptions underpin the very way in which we choose to work with people. As such, they are of pervasive importance to our therapeutic practice, which is all the more surprising – and potentially worrying – when one realises just how few people really have given any sustained consideration to these issues of what, in their view, constitutes the fundamentals of human nature. Try the exercise in Box 2.2 as a starting point for reflection on your own views of human nature.

This issue is especially true, we believe, for trainee clinical psychologists and other novice therapists, whose training equips them to use a variety of different techniques, but often without reflection on their basic assumptions. To practise as a therapist we must surely hold that people have the capacity for change. We must also reflect on our assumptions about how change is possible. The deep-seated assumptions of a therapist are seen in their choice of words. When asked about their practice, one therapist will talk about getting the client to move on, another will talk about their task being to understand the client's history, yet another will talk about their management of the client's symptoms. Each is giving a taste of his or her own views of human nature, and about how those views fundamentally influence them in their practice of striving to help another person. In those contexts where all share similar views, the deep-seated assumptions go unnoticed because there are no points of contrast.

Box 2.2 Exploring your perceptions

The following exercise can be carried out in groups and used to form the basis of discussion to explore differences in perception.
  Read the following questions and then answer whether you think the answer is A, B, or C.

1   When people are selfish, greedy, or unkind is it mostly because . . .?
    A   of the way they were brought up
    B   they were just born that way
    C   of the circumstances in which they are living.
2   When people are loving, kind, and generous, is it mostly because . . .?
    A   of the way they were brought up
    B   they were just born that way
    C   of the circumstances in which they are living.

When a therapist talks about getting their client to 'move on', there is the message that it is the therapist, and not the client, who is the expert and who knows best as to how to proceed. This message stands in stark contrast to those other therapeutic approaches that hold that it is the client and not the therapist who is the best expert on themselves.

When a therapist talks about the need to understand the client's history, there is the message that this is important and useful in order to help the client. This message stands in stark contrast to those therapeutic approaches which hold that although early history might be important in understanding how problems have arisen, it is not necessary to unravel these in order for the client to make new choices in their life.

Similarly, when we talk about the management of 'symptoms', there is the message that the client's problems are symptomatic of some so-called psychological disorder, as opposed to them experiencing problems of living, in which no judgement of normality versus abnormality is required.

We want to emphasise that any practice of psychology rests on our fundamental assumptions about human nature. These assumptions may be deep seated, but they are also easily seen in our choice of words. Our assumptions as therapists will reflect our own personalities and preferences, forged through our own life experiences and therapeutic training. These assumptions do not lend themselves to straightforward empirical inquiry, and hence may be considered as questions of value and morality – and thus individual ethics and preference. Further, these assumptions are typically implicit, and therefore are often uncritically accepted by practitioners trained in a particular model and a particular way of working. It is precisely because these fundamental assumptions are implicit that they are so often taken for granted and unchallenged, assuming the position of the status quo. Importantly, these fundamental assumptions are inevitably formed within a particular social, cultural, and historical context (cf. Marcus & Fischer, 1986; Prilleltensky, 1994). This social, cultural, and historical boundedness, fixed as it is to a particular place and time, may limit the relevance of the fundamental assumptions formed within it as times change. We will elaborate more on this below, but first let us turn to the assumptions themselves.

Martin Seligman and positive psychology

Having emphasised how practice rests on what are often implicit and rarely articulated fundamental assumptions, we want to articulate and make explicit these assumptions. Broadly speaking, our view of human nature falls into one of two camps: either that human nature is basically negative and destructive, or that it is positive and constructive. It has been suggested that the fundamental assumptions of mainstream psychology are those of the former. As Martin Seligman, the champion of positive psychology, has said:

> There has been a profound obstacle to a science and practice of positive traits and positive states: the belief that virtue and happiness are inauthentic, epiphenomenal, parasitic upon or reducible to the negative traits and states. This 'rotten-to-the-core' view pervades Western thought, and if there is any doctrine positive psychology seeks to overthrow it is this one. Its original manifestation is the doctrine of original sin. In secular form, Freud dragged this doctrine into 20th-century psychology where it remains fashionably entrenched in academia today. For Freud, all of civilization is just an elaborate defence against basic conflicts over infantile sexuality and aggression.
>
> (Seligman, 2003a, p. 126)

As Seligman (2002, 2003a) notes, much of modern psychology has been dominated by the doctrines of Freud, 'the ghost in the machine' of psychology and psychotherapy (Hubble & Miller, 2004). Positive psychology has made explicit the fact that psychology has traditionally rested on a fundamental assumption that emphasises human nature as negative in orientation and needing to be controlled (see Hubble & Miller, 2004; Maddux, 2002; Maddux et al., 2004b). If Seligman is right and this view pervades Western academic thought, then we must accept that much of what goes on in the name of professional psychology is about 'cutting out the rotten bits'.

Yet rarely do psychologists stop and reflect on where and why this view arose. Is it true that people are 'rotten-to-the-core'? We will argue that the evidence just does not point this way, and although it is true that people inflict much pain and suffering on each other, there are other explanations for this that do not require us to adopt the assumption that people are 'rotten-to-the-core'.

If positive psychology as a discipline rejects the 'rotten-to-the-core' view of human nature, what is the alternative? Implicit within positive psychology is the idea that human beings have the potential for 'good', and that we are motivated to pursue a 'good life'. Thus, our implicit notion of value and morality requires that positive psychology's fundamental assumption about human nature take account of these implicit values (the potential for 'good' and the desire for a 'good life'). Having discarded the 'rotten-to-the-core' view of human nature, positive psychologists are now casting around for new ways to conceptualise human nature. Fortunately, psychology has a very rich heritage of ideas, and when we look into the past of our discipline we find that the questions we are now asking are ones that many of the greatest psychologists have also tackled. One of the first psychologists to make the nature of our fundamental assumptions explicit was Karen Horney.

Karen Horney and the morality of evolution

In considering how views of human nature influenced our perspective on the promotion of living a good life (or a *morality of evolution*), Horney (1951) delineated three possible positions in trying to understand core human nature. The first position was that people are by nature sinful or driven by primitive instincts. This first perspective accords with the 'rotten-to-the-core' view that we have just discussed. The second position was that inherent within human nature was both something essentially 'good' and something essentially 'bad', sinful, or destructive. From this second position, the goal of society is to ensure that the 'good' side of human nature triumphs over the 'bad' side. The third position was that inherent within people are evolutionary constructive forces that guide people towards realising their potentialities. Horney was careful to note that this third position did *not* suggest that people were inherently good (since this would presuppose knowledge of what constitutes good and bad). Rather, the person's values would arise from their striving towards their potential, and these values would thus be constructive and prosocial in their nature (and hence may be considered 'good'). From this third position, the goal of society is therefore to cultivate the facilitative social–environmental conditions that are conducive to people's self-realisation. When people's tendency toward self-realisation is allowed expression, Horney argued that:

> [W]e become free to grow ourselves, we also free ourselves to love and to feel concern for other people. We will then want to give them the opportunity for unhampered growth when they are young, and to help them in whatever way possible to find and realize themselves when they are blocked in their development. At any rate, whether for ourselves or for others, the ideal is the liberation and cultivation of the forces which lead to self-realization.
>
> (Horney, 1951, pp. 15–16)

Carl Rogers and the actualising tendency

Horney was not the only psychologist to reach this conclusion. The most influential of all the psychologists who adopted this perspective was Carl Rogers (see Thorne, 1992 for a biography) who almost 50 years ago was asking the same questions as positive psychologists are today. Like Seligman, Carl Rogers questioned the fundamental assumptions of mainstream psychology in his day, proposing instead the view that human beings are organismically motivated toward developing their full potential:

I have little sympathy with the rather prevalent concept that man is basically irrational, and thus his impulses, if not controlled, would lead to destruction of others and self. Man's behavior is exquisitely rational, moving with subtle and ordered complexity toward the goals his organism is endeavoring to achieve.

(Rogers, 1969, p. 29)

This is similar to Horney's third position just discussed. Deep within us, Rogers proposed, human beings are striving to become all that they can be. Rogers referred to this directional force of becoming as the *actualising tendency*:

This is the inherent tendency of the organism to develop all its capacities in ways which serve to maintain or enhance the organism. It involves not only the tendency to meet what Maslow terms 'deficiency needs' for air, food, water, and the like, but also more generalized activities. It involves development toward the differentiation of organs and of functions, expansion in terms of growth, expansion of effectiveness through the use of tools, expansion and enhancement through reproduction. It is development toward autonomy and away from heteronomy, or control by external forces.

(Rogers, 1959, p. 196)

Rogers (1959) was conceptualising the basic directionality of the actualising tendency as toward the development of autonomous determination, expansion and effectiveness, and constructive social behaviour. The actualising tendency, Rogers argued, was the one natural motivational force of human beings, one is always directed towards constructive growth.

It is the urge which is evident in all organic and human life – to expand, extend, to become autonomous, develop, mature – the tendency to express and activate all the capacities of the organism, to the extent that such activation enhances the organism or the self.

(Rogers, 1961, p. 35)

To vividly illustrate the concept, Rogers described how during a vacation he was overlooking one of the rugged coves that dot the coastline of northern California:

Several large rock outcroppings were at the mouth of the cove, and these received the full force of the great pacific combers which, beating upon them, broke into mountains of spray before surging into the cliff-lined shore. As I watched the waves breaking over these large rocks in the distance, I noticed with surprise what appeared to be tiny palm trees on the rocks, no more than two or three feet high, taking the pounding of the breakers. Through my binoculars I saw that these were some type of seaweed, with a slender 'trunk' topped off with a head of leaves. As one examined a specimen in the intervals between the waves it seemed clear that this fragile, erect, top-heavy plant would be utterly crushed and broken by the next breaker. When the wave crunched down upon it, the trunk bent almost flat, the leaves were whipped into a straight line by the torrent of water, yet the moment the wave had passed, here was the plant again, erect, tough, resilient . . . Here in this palmlike seaweed was the tenacity of life, the forward thrust of life, the ability to push into an incredibly hostile environment and not only hold its own, but to adapt, develop, and become itself.

(Rogers, 1961, pp. 1–2)

Rogers used this example of how all organisms, be they palmlike seaweed or people, can be counted on to be directed toward maintaining, enhancing, and reproducing. The actualising tendency is thought to be the basic and sole motivation of people. The actualising tendency is a universal motivation always resulting in growth, development, and autonomy of the individual. In writing about the actualising tendency, Rogers (1963a) states:

We are, in short, dealing with an organism which is always motivated, is always 'up to something', always seeking. So I would reaffirm, perhaps even more strongly after the passage of a decade, my belief that there is one central source of energy in the human organism; that it is a function of the whole organism rather than some portion of it; and that it is best conceptualized as a tendency toward fulfilment, toward actualization, toward the maintenance and enhancement of the organism.

(Rogers, 1963a, p. 6)

The actualising tendency as a fundamental assumption about human nature

Within the history of psychology, Karen Horney and Carl Rogers are two of the proponents of the fundamental assumption about human nature that posits a constructive directional tendency. However, Horney and Rogers were not the only psychologists to discuss this perspective on human nature. Other well-known theorists who have proposed some form of actualising tendency include Adler (1927), Angyal (1941), Goldstein (1939), Jung (1933), Maslow (1968), and Rank (1936).

Also, as we shall see in later chapters, it is an idea that has found favour with other contemporary positive psychologists, such as Deci and Ryan (2000) who in their theory of self-determination also propose that people are intrinsically motivated towards optimal functioning. Thus, the concept of an actualising tendency has a distinguished heritage in psychology and resonance in contemporary positive psychology.

We have argued elsewhere (Linley & Joseph, 2004c) that this fundamental assumption of the tendency towards actualisation promises to provide the central theoretical foundation stone for the new science of positive psychology, and for what we call positive therapy (Joseph & Linley, 2004, 2005). These perspectives proposed by Horney and Rogers agree that there is a constructive developmental tendency within human nature, and that this tendency, when given appropriate expression, leads to the well-being of both the individual and their wider community and society. These theories are also consistent in the way in which they each account for ill-being or psychopathology, suggesting that ill-being and psychopathology arise to the extent that the individual has lost contact with their innate directional force.

This is, we would argue, one of the 'big ideas' of psychology, but one that has been largely forgotten about in contemporary psychology. As we shall go on to discuss throughout this book, the implication of this big idea for professional psychological practice is that the client knows best. When we say this we know a common criticism is that if the client knows best what are they coming to therapy for? But this is to misunderstand the idea. It is not that people can easily articulate their best directions in life, but with the right support they can begin to work out for themselves solutions to their own problems. It can be seen in the attitude of any therapist whether they view themselves as the expert on their client or whether they view their client as their own best expert.

The client as their own best expert

Carl Rogers developed an approach to professional practice called the person-centred approach, which embraces this idea – that people are their own best experts. This is a general philosophical approach to working with people that can be applied in a variety of settings, with individuals, couples, groups, and organisations. In this book, we are concerned with the therapeutic setting and the face-to-face encounter of two people. We will go on in Chapter 4 to describe client-centred therapy in more detail, but for the moment we want to illustrate how a therapeutic approach founded on the assumption of an actualising tendency leads to the idea that the client knows best.

Rogers emphasised that it was how the individual perceives reality that was important and that the best vantage point for understanding a person is that person. In this respect, Rogers ideas resonate well with the ideas of cognitive therapy. However, although cognitive therapy also emphasises that it is how the person perceives reality that is important in shaping psychopathology, cognitive therapy does not necessarily adopt the view that it is the client who knows best what direction to take. Some cognitive-behavioural therapists will work in a person-centred way, but others will work in a more traditional medical model way. In working in the medical model way, the therapist adopts the assumption that it is he or she that knows best, and who will direct the client in the direction that he or she believes is best for the client. The therapist is there to show the client a different way to look at their situation, to show the client new possibilities, to teach new ways of thinking, to direct the client to techniques for stopping anxious thoughts, to learn how to relax when feeling stressed, and so on. There is the assumption that people need some direction from the therapist because they do not have it within them to know what their own best directions in life are. The client is not the best expert on himself or herself; the *therapist* is their best expert. Insofar as therapy is akin to the practice of medicine this idea is not strange. After all, if we break our leg we do need help from someone who is more expert than us to help us know what to do. But we argue that much of what psychologists, psychotherapists, and counsellors do is not actually akin to the practice of medicine, but is instead about facilitating a person to listen to their own inner wisdom. Thus, the person is his or her own best expert.

When the therapist is working on this assumption that people know, deep within themselves, what is best for them, the task of the therapist is to help the client hear their own inner voice. As we shall go on to show, the ideas of Carl Rogers provided a profound and revolutionary approach to professional practice (see Bozarth, 1998). As Brazier put it:

> The bedrock of Rogers' philosophy was the notion that the person is a living experiencing organism whose basic tendencies are trustworthy. It is still difficult for most people in the modern age to appreciate how revolutionary this simple idea is. It is not until we start to consider how much of our energy in modern society is spent on building and maintaining structures, the primary purpose of which is to eliminate the (dangerous) human element from human interactions, that we begin to get a glimpse of how radical Rogers' vision was and still is.
>
> (Brazier, 1993, pp. 7–8)

Challenging the medical model

The ideas of Carl Rogers and the person-centred approach he originated are popular among many counsellors and psychotherapists, but for some reason have become ignored, misunderstood, and disregarded by the profession of psychology (see Joseph, 2003a). There are a variety of possible reasons for this. One reason can be clearly traced from the early history of clinical psychology (Maddux et al., 2004b). Early clinical psychology training took place in psychiatric hospitals and clinics under the supervision of psychiatrists who were trained in medicine and psychoanalysis, thus permeating the fledgling profession of clinical psychology with the illness ideology and the medical model. Subsequently, in the United States, the establishment of the Veterans Administration after World War II created training centres and standards for clinical psychologists, but which were again steeped in the tradition of psychiatrists. Further, the founding of the United States National Institute of Mental Health channelled millions of research dollars toward the understanding and treatment of mental illness, thus further influencing the direction in which clinical psychology evolved (Maddux et al., 2004b). These developments allowed a rise in status for the profession of clinical psychology, but one that required its adoption of the illness ideology and the medical model, so as to maintain consistency with its psychiatric masters (Maddux et al., 2004b). As such, clinical psychology evolved largely as a profession that exists not to facilitate potential, but, as Brazier (1993) puts it, to eliminate the dangerous human element.

We believe that the medical model and the illness ideology are simply the wrong way to think about human distress and psychological suffering, and that those who adopt the medical model and the illness ideology damage their clients, and impede their potential for optimal functioning (see Sanders, 2005). However, we also recognise that the medical model has become widely accepted among psychologists, and that it will take some time to extricate the profession of clinical psychology and reorient it toward a more productive framework for understanding psychopathology and well-being. However, movements toward a positive clinical psychology are doing just that (Maddux et al., 2004b), and as we shall go on to show in Chapter 6, positive psychology is infusing powerful new ways of thinking about psychopathology and well-being into approaches to what has been called 'positive clinical psychology' (Maddux et al., 2004b; Peterson & Seligman, 2003). Importantly, these positive clinical psychology models provide a new way of approaching the clinical psychology paradigm that is in keeping with the meta-theoretical position of the actualising tendency that we have described, and as such, offer the potential for a radical new integration of the ideas of person-centred theory, positive psychology, and mainstream clinical psychology (see Chapter 6). We are also profoundly encouraged that younger members of the profession are being drawn to the new ideas of the positive psychology movement, and when we look to the future we now see hope for change.

We think the ideas of Carl Rogers have now come of age with the dawning of the positive psychology movement. We think it is refreshing for our profession that positive psychology has provided the impetus for us to now reexamine our fundamental assumptions about human nature, particularly with regard to the medical model, and the actualising tendency as the core motivational force for optimal human development. We will come back to these themes again in Chapter 6, when we discuss our understanding of psychopathology.

The meaning of well-being

We will go on to argue that the fundamental assumption of an inherent actualising tendency provides the foundation for a positive therapy. But first, it is important to consider the question of what is good and desirable within positive psychology. Often, our assumptions about what is good and desirable are also implicit rather than explicit and we think that it is vital that we are also reflective of these assumptions.

The value assumptions implicit within positive psychology are also fundamental for the prescriptions we make on what are good and desirable. Especially as attention moves from basic research to practice, and the science of positive psychology moves from being descriptive to prescriptive, these values critically inform the directions that our interventions and facilitative work takes. Again, it is worth noting at this point that this position is no different than that of any other applied psychology discipline. Just as all clinical psychology, counselling psychology, and industrial/organisational psychology operate from a (typically implicit) value position, so too does applied positive psychology, and positive therapy. Our intention here, however, is to render this value position explicit, and hence open to scrutiny, criticism, and revision as appropriate.

Seligman (e.g., Seligman, 2002; Seligman & Csikszentmihalyi, 2000) has defined the 'desired outcomes' (i.e., valued goods) of positive psychology as happiness and well-being. This could be taken to suggest that in any value hierarchy within positive psychology, happiness and well-being would be found at the head of such a hierarchy. However, we suggest that this was not necessarily Seligman's intent, and we will go on to demonstrate why. What we need to do is to reflect on what we mean when we talk of well-being.

First, what is meant by 'happiness' and 'well-being' is crucial. If our 'happiness' is to be found, for example, through exploiting others, is that a legitimate aim for positive psychology and for positive therapy? Of course it is not, and Seligman and Csikszentmihalyi (2000) address this through reference to what they term 'collective well-being'. Hence, implicitly, the further value position is adopted that the happiness and well-being of any given individual should not be at the detriment and cost of others. Indeed, if it were, how would one decide who merited happiness, and who merited suffering for that person's happiness? These questions concern the first of the three levels of positive psychology, that is, valued subjective experiences. Hence, we may have valued subjective experiences that are not in keeping with the third level of positive civic virtues, such as civility, tolerance, and responsibility. If anything, these may restrain our happiness. However, here the definition of happiness is crucial. An important distinction for understanding well-being is that between what is referred to as psychological well-being (PWB) and subjective well-being (SWB).

Psychological well-being and subjective well-being

Psychological well-being and subjective well-being are derived from two general philosophical perspectives, the eudaemonic and the hedonic approach (see Ryan & Deci, 2001). The well-being described by Horney and Rogers is also captured much more fully by the concept of psychological well-being. Indeed, throughout the psychological literature, a number of authors have drawn this distinction both empirically (Compton, Smith, Cornish, & Qualls, 1996; Keyes, Shmotkin, & Ryff, 2002; McGregor & Little, 1998; Ryff, 1989; Waterman, 1993) and theoretically (Ryan & Deci, 2001; Ryff & Singer, 1996). This distinction has important implications for positive psychology, and especially applied positive psychology and positive therapy.

Happiness defined within the scientific term of subjective well-being is the sum of life satisfaction and affective balance (i.e., positive affect minus negative affect). In this regard, Seligman and Csikszentmihalyi (2000) raised the issue of 'the calculus of well-being' – what can we do to be consistently happier? Yet, as Kahneman (1999) notes, this may be largely impossible (but see Sheldon & Lyubomirsky, 2004, for a contrasting perspective; see Seligman et al., 2005, for preliminary data showing that happiness can be increased). However, what would it mean if positive psychology had been looking at the wrong type of happiness? There may be much merit to the argument that increases in happiness are unsustainable because of the 'hedonic treadmill' (Brickman & Campbell, 1971). This accords with much of the research evidence.

In contrast, psychological well-being (defined as 'engagement with the existential challenges of life'; Keyes et al., 2002) provides a much broader and more rounded context of well-being. It is also more fully compatible with the positive psychological functioning that results from acting congruently with one's organismic valuing process, a topic that we will discuss more fully in Chapter 3.

The implications of these different types of well-being for applied positive psychology and positive therapy are important. First, as we noted, the 'calculus of well-being' does not suggest how happiness may be sustainably increased – in contrast, much of the research evidence points to the transitory and fleeting nature of this subjective experience (Kahneman, 1999). Even Sheldon and Lyubomirsky's (2004) work on sustainable boosts in happiness, and Seligman and colleagues' (2005) findings are characterised, we suggest, by activities that are more in keeping with a psychological well-being perspective (i.e., practising gratitude, performing acts of kindness) than a strictly subjective well-being perspective. Although the two types of well-being are typically moderately correlated (Compton et al., 1996; Keyes et al., 2002; Waterman, 1993), this should not be taken to mean that they are largely synonymous. Important distinctions arise between people who have much pleasure in life but are unfulfilled (i.e., high SWB, low PWB) and between people who may not be perceived as 'happy' but who find their lives deeply meaningful (even in the context of chronic suffering) (i.e., low SWB, high PWB). Such people have been described as 'off-diagonal' (Keyes et al., 2002), since in their instances the correlations between SWB and PWB do not hold. One may also consider such people within Seligman's (2002) theory of authentic happiness: the pleasant life may be characterised by physical pleasure but the absence of fulfilment and growth (e.g., high SWB, low PWB), whereas the meaningful life combines both pleasure and a higher meaning and fulfilment, working in the service of something greater than oneself (high SWB, high PWB).

Implications of the SWB–PWB distinction for practice

The implications of the distinction for practice are considerable. If SWB were the goal of applied positive psychology and positive therapy, should we sanction ever greater experience of momentary positive affect and avoidance of negative affect? On this basis, ever more consumption and greater luxury should serve to boost our momentary hedonic states. Yet, the evidence clearly indicates the contrary: more money, more materialism, and more possessions all singularly fail to make us any happier (Csikszentmihalyi, 1999; Kasser, 2002; Myers, 2000). In contrast, they may have even the reverse effect, leading to psychological ill-being (Kasser, 2004; Kasser & Ryan, 1993, 1996) and greater ecological costs that are a detriment to our long-term environmental well-being and survival (Sheldon & McGregor, 2000). We can infer that psychological well-being does not fall prey to the problems of the calculus of well-being as does subjective well-being. There is no hedonic treadmill for PWB, which is more appropriately viewed as an ongoing process rather than a fixed state, whereas SWB is of its nature limited by how much pleasure we can experience at any given passing moment.

Having emphasised these distinctions between SWB and PWB, we suggest that the exclusive pursuit of SWB (i.e., the more common 'happiness') is likely to be a futile and contradictory pursuit. In contrast, PWB, taken as representative of the positive psychological functioning espoused by Horney, and Rogers, is more appropriately adopted as a desired outcome of positive psychology. What all these conceptions have in common, and which is implicit within the concept of PWB, is its location in the context of the individual within community and culture, rather than the individual in isolation.

Thus, PWB as we understand it, and as we propose it within the positive therapy approach, is concerned as much with collective well-being as it is with individual well-being. In this way, PWB can be seen as at the head of the applied positive psychology value hierarchy, but not at the expense of civic virtues such as tolerance, civility, and responsibility. Rather, we would argue, PWB could not occur except within a context that respected the 'desired goods' of the third level of positive psychology, positive institutions and civic virtues. This position thus reflects Sternberg's (1998) extrapersonal dimension of wisdom; the value relativism in wisdom as described by Baltes (e.g., Baltes & Staudinger, 2000; Baltes, Gluck, & Kunzmann, 2002); and the permanent adversities (i.e., contingency, conflict, and plurality within values) that inhibit the path to the good life described by Kekes (1995).

When well-being as a desired outcome of positive psychology is made explicit and conceptualised in this way, it is more fully consistent with the fuller understanding of the goals of applied positive psychology and positive therapy. This more easily allows their interrelationships to be documented and understood, rather than being seen as inconsistent and potentially incompatible. In essence, the pursuit of ever more subjective well-being is likely to be personally, socially, and environmentally unsustainable (Kahnemen, 1999; Sheldon & McGregor, 2000). However, the pursuit of greater psychological well-being is, we would argue, inbuilt into what it means to be human. Rogers (1961) in discussing 'the good life' wrote:

> It seems to me that the good life is not any fixed state. It is not, in my estimation, a state of virtue, or contentment, or nirvana, or happiness. It is not a condition in which the individual is adjusted, fulfilled, or actualized . . . The good life is a *process*, not a state of being . . . It is a direction, not a destination. The direction . . . is that which is selected by the total organism, when there is psychological freedom to move in *any* direction.
> (Rogers, 1961, pp. 186–187)

The actualising tendency guides us all to ever more development, fulfilment, and integration, and as we set out earlier, this is explicitly a socially constructive force, rather than a selfish, destructive one. It is important to be clear, therefore, that in talking about happiness and well-being as desired outcomes of applied positive psychology and positive therapy, we are talking about psychological well-being, or growth and fulfilment, rather than transitory hits of sensual pleasure.

An integrative view of the human condition

Just as we have emphasised the two approaches to well-being and their implications for positive therapy and practice, so we also emphasise the need for positive therapy to adopt an integrative approach that is encompassing of both the positive and negative aspects of human experience. We do not in any way claim positive therapy as being the preserve of the worried well, or as only being of relevance and use for people who are functioning 'okay' but would like to be functioning 'well' – far from it, as we go on to show in Chapter 6. Importantly within positive psychology, this integration of the positive and negative recognises both sides of the human condition, the experience of positive and negative emotions, which are inescapably part of what it means to be human (Linley & Joseph, 2003). We do not wish to negate or do away with psychology's attention to suffering and distress, but rather to locate them within the context of full human functioning. For example, Larsen, Hemenover, Norris, and Cacioppo (2003) have delineated how the brain systems that underlie positive and negative emotions are distinct but may also be coactivated. This coactivation may be experienced as unstable, unpleasant, and disharmonious, but it may be key to working through and transcending major life stressors: in essence, one must be able to confront adversity, but also accept and find meaning in it.

In a similar vein, Ryff and Singer (2003) describe how good lives are effortful and challenging, and arise from zest and engagement in living. Thus, for a life to be considered good, it would not be characterised by an easy pleasure, but rather by an active and determined quest to overcome obstacles, to live being mindful of our mortality, and appreciating life therefore all the more. It is for this reason that we (e.g., Linley & Joseph, 2002a, 2002b, 2002c) have referred to posttraumatic growth as the 'apotheosis of positive psychology'. Posttraumatic growth represents the PWB after which positive psychology aspires, but within a context of suffering and adversity that debunks any criticism of positive psychology's 'Pollyanna theorising' (cf. Linley & Joseph, 2004c; Linley, Joseph, Cooper, Harris, & Meyer, 2003). Hence, in integrating the positive and the negative within the context of posttraumatic growth, we have described a tragic hopefulness that encapsulates both recognition of our existential position and inevitable mortality, and described how wisdom may be one positive outcome of the struggle with trauma (Linley, 2003). Despite this, we still maintain a desire to live and grow, and make the most of what we have (Linley, 2000; Linley & Joseph, 2002a, 2002b, 2002c).

Positive psychology and the nature of knowledge

Just as positive psychology has challenged us to consider our fundamental assumptions about human nature, and positive therapy challenges us to consider our beliefs about ourselves as artists or scientists, so too does positive psychology raise our awareness about questions of epistemology and the nature of knowledge. From the outset, Seligman (e.g., 2001) has striven to ensure that positive psychology is a discipline characterised by good empirical science. This is a position that we support, and fully agree that scientific pedigree should be a hallmark of positive psychology research and practice. However, we must also be mindful about the nature of the questions that we are asking. In considering the ideas discussed earlier about human nature and assumptions that we adopt, we are left with questions of values (which are relative) and morality (which is a matter of personal ethics). Neither of these can be scientifically proven right or wrong, since they are not empirical questions per se, but rather reflect the standpoint from which we have chosen to operate. Hence, while the empirical method has taught us much, and guards against conjecture and anecdote being accepted in place of scientific research, we must be aware that it cannot tell us everything. Some questions, quite simply, are irreducible to empirical questions that fit neat experimental methodologies.

Positive psychology and the limits of empirical science

These caveats notwithstanding, advances in our methodological and statistical knowledge do allow important questions to be answered with a degree of empirical sophistication that was not previously possible. Hence, it is not our intention at all to suggest that the non-empirical nature of some of these questions be used as an excuse for 'bad science' – far from it. We only wish to note that empirical methodologies may not be equipped to answer all our questions of interest, and hence we should be receptive to a variety of methods of inquiry, being careful to recognise the appropriate place and value of each.

For example, relatively recent developments in experience sampling methodologies and diary studies have been used to lend greater validity to self-report data. The growing array of qualitative methodologies (e.g., interpretative phenomenological analysis, grounded theory, discourse analysis) have already allowed us insights into aspects of human experience that would not have been detected through directive questionnaires or artificial laboratory settings. (See Larsen et al., 2003, for an example of the coactivation of positive and negative affect that was detected only through using an experience sampling methodology.)

Human experience is at the core of much positive psychology, and as Rathunde (2001) notes, researchers could learn much from the 'experiential turns' of such early psychological pioneers as Dewey, James, and Maslow, who focused on immediate subjective experience in trying to understand optimal human fulfilment. In seeking to objectify psychology in the positivist scientific tradition, Rathunde argues that many rich data from subjective experience have been unnecessarily excluded from psychological discourse. It would be eminently regrettable, we believe, if this were allowed to continue.

The questions that positive psychology and the practice of positive psychology lead us to ask may be beyond the remit of our current experimental designs and abilities. However, we should not thereby exclude the questions as not worth asking, but should rather seek to answer them in the most appropriate way that we can. Our guiding ethos should not be which questions fit with our scientific methods, but what methods, scientific or otherwise, may be most appropriate for answering the questions of interest to us. These are far from issues that will be easily resolved, but the questions are fundamental as we develop the further practice of positive psychology and positive therapy.

Conclusion

In this chapter, we have raised what we see as some fundamental issues for the practice of positive psychology and positive therapy. These issues challenge us as psychologists and as practitioners to be reflective of the way we work with people, and equally importantly, of the 'why' we work with people in the way we do. We have raised the question of whether as therapists we prefer to see ourselves as artistes or scientists, and what the implications of our choice are for the way in which we work with our clients.

We have addressed the question of fundamental assumptions about human nature, showing how, in broad terms, we may adopt one of three positions: that people are intrinsically motivated by destructive impulses that need to be controlled; that people may be motivated by either destructive or constructive impulses and we should therefore control the destructive and facilitate the constructive; or that people are by nature motivated by positive, constructive directional tendencies toward the actualisation of their potentialities. We have argued that positive psychology and positive therapy adopt this third position, and we have started to show how these principles can be traced back to the work of Carl Rogers and person-centred theory, to which we turn more fully in Chapter 3.

Finally, we have raised some challenging questions for positive psychology and the practice of positive therapy, examining the desired outcomes or valued goods of positive psychology, and exploring the distinction between psychological and subjective conceptions of well-being and their implications for practice. We also highlighted the importance of open reflection on these issues, including the need for an integrative approach to the human condition, and a recognition of the epistemological limits of a scientific positive psychology and an empirical positive therapy. These are deeply challenging philosophical issues, and rather than provide answers, we simply sought to raise awareness of them and their implication for positive therapeutic practice, that therapists might be able to reflect actively on what they mean for their ways of working with people. In the next chapter, we build on these topics to explore more fully the ideas of Carl Rogers and person-centred theory, and elucidate how this therapeutic approach provides a solid theoretical foundation and a rich historical lineage to the more recent development of positive therapy.

Chapter 3

The organismic valuing process and person-centred theories

As we discussed in Chapter 2, therapists do, whether it is to give advice, interpret, reassure, listen, ask questions, or whatever else, is contextualised by their view of human nature. What we began to do in Chapter 2 was to show the paradigmatic difference that can exist between therapists, depending on their fundamental assumptions about human nature. Broadly speaking, we either view human nature as destructive or constructive. Furthermore, we began to illustrate how an individual's approach to the artistry of therapy inevitably follows on from their view of human nature. Two therapists are listening to their client talk. To an outside observer both just look as if they are listening. But depending on their fundamental assumptions they may be listening in very different ways indeed. As already mentioned, if people's nature is essentially driven by destructive impulses, then the role of the therapists is to help keep tight the constraints on those impulses. If people's nature is essentially driven by constructive impulses, then our role is to loosen the constraints on those impulses. Those two therapists are listening in very different ways indeed.

In the previous chapter we briefly introduced the person-centred approach of Carl Rogers. In this chapter, we will describe Rogers' (1959) person-centred personality theory in more detail. In particular, we will introduce the concept of the organismic valuing process, that is, people's innate ability to know what is important to them and what is essential for a fulfilling life. Then we will examine contemporary positive psychology theory showing how there are current trends that have a lineage to person-centred theory, and how current research evidence in positive psychology is supportive of the basic premises of person-centred personality theory.

Carl Rogers and the person-centred approach

Before we describe person-centred theory, we wish to say a little about its founder, Carl Rogers. Although today Rogers is best remembered for his work in introducing the field of counselling, Rogers was originally a psychologist by training. Indeed, at one point in his career he even served as the President of the American Psychological Association. He had many achievements in his life, one of the earliest of which was to pioneer psychotherapy research. Rogers was the first psychologist to use recordings of therapeutic sessions for research (Rogers, 1942), and by listening back to the therapy sessions, Rogers and his colleagues were the first to examine what actually went on during therapy.

Throughout his life Rogers was a prolific writer, publishing numerous academic papers and books, many of which are still widely read today. In his book *Client-Centered Therapy*, Rogers began to outline his model of counselling and psychotherapy (Rogers, 1951). Rogers used the terms counselling and psychotherapy interchangeably, only introducing the term counselling early in his career because of objections raised by the profession of psychiatry to his use of the term psychotherapy. At the time, psychotherapy was seen as the province of psychiatry and medicine, and Rogers, as a psychologist, was therefore not seen to be able to offer psychotherapy. Of course, this situation has changed today, and psychologists regularly practise counselling and psychotherapy. Because of this terminological heritage, some still view counselling as associated with client-centred therapy and psychotherapy as associated with psychoanalysis. However, consistent with the person-centred approach we use the terms interchangeably in this book with the term therapy.

After the publication of *Client-Centered Therapy*, Rogers went on to describe his ideas in more detail in later papers as he elaborated on his theory of personality and therapy (Rogers, 1957, 1959). Over the years, Rogers began to apply his ideas derived from therapy in wider contexts, such as education, conflict resolution, and encounter groups (see Thorne, 1992). In order to recognise the broader applicability of his model the term person centred came to replace the term client centred. These terms are often used interchangeably, although some prefer to use the term client centred when referring to therapeutic work, and the term person centred when referring to the broader applications of the theory. When one reads the writings of Rogers on the broader applicability of person-centred theory, the lineage of positive psychology can be easily seen (see Barrett-Lennard, 1998; Kirschenbaum & Henderson, 1989).

Sometimes client-centred therapy is referred to as Rogerian therapy. However, Rogers disliked the use of this term maintaining that he did not want to see a school of therapists who were modelling themselves on him but rather to see therapists who were able to find their own ways of working within the person-centred approach. However, although the early development of the client-centred tradition was fuelled by the results of scientific inquiry, later in his career Rogers moved away from working in academic psychological settings and as a result the person-centred approach became less of a focus for research attention. This was the time of the 1960s and 1970s and the encounter group movement. As a result, when many people think of person-centred psychology, they think back to this time, rather than to the earlier, more academic context in which the theory remains firmly rooted (Rogers, 1957, 1959). It seems to us that person-centred theory is a theory of human nature that has remained constant, while the contexts in which the theory is applied have continued to change, a point that, we would argue, speaks to the lasting durability of its central propositions. Both the early scientific client-centred movement and the later person-centred and encounter group traditions are valid in their different ways, and there is much that can be learned from both.

Meanwhile, within academic psychological settings of the 1970s, the cognitive-behavioural approach was gaining in popularity and attracting the interest of clinical research scientists. While proponents of the person-centred approach had turned their attention to experiential learning and new ways of living, academic psychologists were continuing to develop their empirical research into the new cognitive-behavioural methods of therapy. These cognitive-behavioural approaches readily lend themselves to 'manualisation' and the 'scientific method'; they can be easily transposed into a 'what to do cookbook' for conducting therapy, an approach that easily lends itself to the scientific hallmarks of objectivity and replication. In contrast, the crux of client-centred therapy is the therapeutic relationship, and since the development of a therapeutic relationship within the therapy setting is much less amenable to objectification and systematic replication, client-centred therapy proved a more challenging test to the methods of scientific psychotherapy research of the time. This led to a growing interest in psychologists conducting research into cognitive-behavioural therapies, and a related decline in the more difficult task of research into client-centred therapy. The outcomes were clear: cognitive-behavioural therapies were relatively easy to test experimentally, and their research heritage blossomed, while that of client-centred therapy was left behind. However, it is critical to remember that the absence of research support does not, of necessity, imply that client-centred therapy was not effective – rather, it was a reflection of the fact that it had not been subjected to the same empirical scrutiny that cognitive-behavioural techniques had. Indeed, when, more recently, psychologists have been able to systematically compare the two approaches, no differences have been found in their effectiveness (King et al., 2000). However, as a result of these developments, the person-centred approach began to be left behind in the research literature, and as the 1980s and 1990s progressed the person-centred movement began to be seen as a historical footnote in the development of psychology.

The person-centred approach has, as a result, been less subject to research in recent years than some other treatments, notably those from the cognitive-behavioural approach (Bozarth & Brodley, 1984), for the reasons we have already described. Today the person-centred approach is less likely to be a treatment of choice for many clients (see also Bohart, O'Hara, & Leitner, 1998). Also, many of those who became interested in the person-centred approach were not only less interested in conducting empirical research into the effectiveness of the therapy, but took the view that an empirical approach was inappropriate, preferring instead phenomenological methods. Although qualitative methods have gained academic respectability over the last few years and now sit comfortably alongside quantitative methods, it was not always so. For many years there was much debate over the relative values of each approach, and qualitative methods were not always accepted within psychology as equal to quantitative methods. Humanistic psychologists emphasised people's unique experiences and adopting phenomenological methods was often seen as anti-scientific and not taken seriously within academic psychology and psychiatry (see DeCarvalho, 1991). Thus, the influence of humanistic psychology waned.

Nevertheless, the approach remains popular within the fields of counselling and psychotherapy (see Joseph & Worsley, 2005a; Kirschenbaum, 2004; Mearns & Thorne, 1999, 2000; Thorne & Lambers, 1998), and with the emergence of the positive psychology movement (Seligman & Csikszentmihalyi, 2000) with its emphasis on scientific practice, we are able to trace the theoretical lineage of positive therapy back to the person-centred personality theory of Carl Rogers, and specifically his development of client-centred therapy.

Person-centred personality theory

We have briefly mentioned client-centred therapy, but it is important to distinguish the therapy (i.e., client-centred therapy) from the theory (i.e., person-centred personality theory) on which it is based. Here we will describe in more detail person-centred personality theory, and some of its key concepts.

The first most important concept is that of the actualising tendency, which we have already described. This is the idea that there is a sole motivational force towards constructive development. As already noted, one criticism of Rogers' theory is that it is too optimistic: if people are so driven by constructive impulses, then why are they so destructive? The theory explains this by saying that although the actualising tendency is the sole motivational force, it becomes thwarted and usurped by conditions of worth that are introjected from external sources.

Conditions of worth

Rogers (1959) was saying that although there is a universal motivational force toward growth and development, this directional force becomes thwarted by our social environment. In person-centred theory, social environments characterised by *conditional positive regard* thwart the organismic valuing process (OVP). An example of conditional positive regard would be when a child interprets from her parent the message that to be loved, she must do well at school. This is not to say that the parents intend harm to their child, perhaps they are simply concerned about her future and want her to do well at school knowing that this will give her more choices later on in life. But the child has a need to be loved, and quickly learns that to receive this love from her parents, she must do well at school. In more extreme cases, the child might live in fear of the school report, knowing that if her parents are not pleased with it she will be scolded. The child internalises this message, that to be loved one must succeed in life, which is said to be a *condition of worth* for her. She grows up learning to value herself only to the extent that she does well at school, and later, that she does well in her career. Many years later, the girl has become an adult, her parents have passed away, and she no longer needs to do well at school (or in her career) in order to please them. However, the message to succeed is so deeply internalised in the psyche of the woman that she accepts it as part of herself. The motivational force to actualise herself has been thwarted and usurped in pursuit of the need to achieve well in her career, and rather than listening to her own inner voice, she is, so to speak, still listening to the voice of her parents that she had internalised in childhood. Thus, as this example demonstrates, conditions of worth are often very subtle. Nevertheless, this subtlety is all the more powerful, since it can render us unaware of what our conditions of worth are, with the influence being much more subtle and lasting far longer than might ostensibly appear to be the case.

Central to the theory is the assumption that we have a need to be positively regarded, and will seek regard from our social environment. If all that is on offer is conditional regard, then that is what we reach out for. For most of us, we grow up with a mix of unconditional and conditional regard from the world around us. We all grow up surrounded by conditions of worth, which we receive from our parents or other carers, teachers and religious educators, media and television, and so on. All these messages tell us about what is important in life, and what we must do to be valued. All of us introject conditions of worth, and to varying extents self-actualise in the direction of our conditions of worth. None of us is fully able to escape the influences of the world around us. Some people's conditions of worth are held so strongly that the actualising tendency becomes thwarted and usurped, so that the person self-actualises in a direction consistent with their conditions of worth as opposed to the actualising tendency.

When self-actualisation is incongruent with the actualising tendency, then psychopathology is evident. For example, in Chapter 2, the reader was introduced to John, who wanted to study writing, but had pursued a career in accountancy under the advice of his parents. John's conditions of worth were to do well at school and although he grew up to be successful in his career, he felt that something was not quite right, he did not enjoy his work, and as he began to listen more closely to himself he began to realise that deep within himself the values he was living were not his but those of his parents, or at least the messages that he had introjected as a young boy about what was important. Throughout his adult life he had tried to live to these values that he had internalised in childhood, and although successful in his career his satisfaction with life was low, and he was often irritable with those around him, and depressed in his mood. What was important to him he began to realise were things he had left behind in childhood, his freedom of expression and his creativity, as he remembered the pleasure and fulfilment he achieved through writing.

Thus, the theory dictates that in a social environment characterised by conditional positive regard, people will self-actualise not in a direction consistent with their actualising tendency, but because of their need for positive regard will self-actualise in a direction consistent with their conditions of worth:

> This, as we see it, is the basic estrangement in man. He has not been true to himself, to his natural organismic valuing of experience, but for the sake of preserving the positive regard of others has now come to falsify some of the values he experiences and to perceiving them in terms based only on their value to others. Yet this has not been a conscious choice, but a natural – and tragic – development in infancy.
>
> (Rogers, 1959, p. 226)

What person-centred theory says is that when the social environment is characterised by *unconditional positive regard*, the child is able to learn that he or she is valued with no strings attached. Thus, rather than learn to listen to others about what they have to do to get love, they learn to listen to themselves. When this happens we can say that self-actualisation and the actualising tendency are coordinated, and that there is a 'unitary actualising tendency' (Rogers, 1963a, p. 20) (see Ford, 1991).

But rarely do we have unconditional positive regard when growing up, and what happens instead is that the positive regard we receive is conditional. In the example of John, he learns to work hard at school to please his parents because to do otherwise would result in the loss of their regard. This is not to say that John

Table 3.1 Example conditions of worth

- To be successful
- To please others
- To bottle up emotions
- To defer to authority
- To not get angry
- To be grateful for what you have
- To not make a fuss

is aware that this is what he is doing. He has introjected the values of his parents so that he has come to value himself only insofar as he succeeds.

Each of us has our own conditions of worth, to work hard, to please others, to be strong – imagine, if love is withheld from a child when she cries, she gets the message 'in order to be loved, I mustn't cry'. This is what Rogers referred to as conditions of worth. In summary, conditions of worth are those messages we introject from society and those around us about how we should behave if we are to be accepted and valued (see Table 3.1). As a consequence we learn to distort and deny certain experiences so that they fit with our picture of self, and we self-actualise in a way consistent with our conditions of worth rather than our actualising tendency.

It is empowering to understand our own conditions of worth. A simple exercise to help do this is presented in Box 3.1. Of course, the exercise will be used differently for different people, not everyone will have had both parents available to them, and therapists would of course vary the exercise appropriately for the person they were with. The exercise can also be used as part of a group teaching exercise and trainees may find it useful to work in small groups allowing them to discuss their conditions of worth, and to share their experiences.

What is important is for the person to think about the people who were very significant to them when they were growing up, to open up to the deep-seated messages they carry within them about what is important in life. The exercise is used to reflect on how early experiences with your caregivers affected how you are today. Sometimes this can be a very upsetting exercise too and therapists need to be cautious in their use of such exercises.

The concept of conditions of worth has an obvious intuitive appeal, but is it supported by empirical research? The answer is

Box 3.1 Exploring our own conditions of worth

First, it is necessary to get into a state of relaxation.

Then, with your eyes closed, imagine going back to the house of your childhood. Imagine standing there at the front door of the house of your childhood. Now go in, walk into your house; now imagine seeing your father, picture him standing there, he turns towards you, and he says to you: 'Whatever you do in life, you must always . . .' Now finish the sentence. You must always . . . what? Don't think too hard, just say to yourself whatever comes immediately to mind.

Now imagine seeing your mother, picture her standing there, she turns to you and says: 'Whatever you do in life, you must always . . .' Finish the sentence. You must always . . . what?

The exercise is used to reflect on how early experiences with your caregivers affect how you are today. The sort of things that people finish these sentences with include:

- work hard to get what you want
- be nice to people if you don't want them to be cross with you
- listen to what other people tell you to do
- do as you are told
- wash your hands before dinner
- say your prayers if you want God to love you
- say thank you for what you've got
- try hard, even if it's not good enough
- be good
- hit people back
- hide your tears
- be strong
- love your parents no matter what
- remember that I love you no matter what.

In thinking about this exercise, you might have had some sentence completions of your own come to mind. They might be similar to some of the ones listed, or ones that are unique to you. People are often surprised by what this exercise reveals to them; it can be a very powerful exercise in helping people to understand their own conditions of worth.

yes. Research with adolescents has shown evidence consistent with Rogers' view, with those adolescents experiencing greater conditional positive regard being less authentic and exhibiting more false-self behaviour (Harter, Marold, Whitesell, & Cobbs, 1996), and ill-being and resentment of parents (Assor, Roth, & Deci, 2004). Also, as we shall see, there is a wealth of positive psychology literature, which although not using the same terminology, is supportive of the general idea that we internalise values from others, and that our well-being is to a large extent determined by the extent to which we internalise the values of others or are able to follow our own values and interests in an autonomous and authentic way.

Fully functioning

As we have seen, Rogers (1959) held that psychological maladjustment develops through the internalisation of conditions of worth. In contrast, in a social environment characterised by unconditional positive regard, people will self-actualise in a direction consistent with their actualising tendency toward becoming what Rogers referred to as fully functioning human beings:

> The 'fully functioning person' is synonymous with optimal psychological adjustment, optimal psychological maturity, complete congruence, complete openness to experience . . . Since some of these terms sound somewhat static, as though such a person 'had arrived' it should be pointed out that all the characteristics of such a person are *process* characteristics. The fully functioning person would be a person-in-process, a person continually changing.
>
> (Rogers, 1959, p. 235) (see also Rogers, 1963b)

The fully functioning person is someone who is accepting of themselves, values all aspects of themselves – their strengths and their weaknesses, is able to live fully in the present, experiences life as a process, finds purpose and meaning in life, desires authenticity in themselves, others, and societal organisations, values deep trusting relationships and is compassionate toward others, and able to receive compassion from others, and is acceptant that change is necessary and inevitable (see Merry, 1999) (see Table 3.2).

Table 3.2 Characteristics of the fully functioning person

- Be open to experience
- Exhibit no defensiveness
- Be able to interpret experience accurately
- Have a flexible rather than static self-concept open to change through experience
- Trust in his or her own experiencing process and develop values in accordance with that experience
- Have no conditions of worth and experience unconditional self-regard
- Be able to respond to new experiences openly
- Be guided by his or her own valuing process through being fully aware of all experience, without the need for denial or distortion of any of it
- Be open to feedback from his or her environment and make realistic changes resulting from that feedback
- Live in harmony with others and experience the rewards of mutual positive regard

The fully functioning person, however, is an ideal. All of us have, to varying extents, self-actualised incongruently to our actualising tendency. For some, incongruence is minimum, for others more substantial, and the more we struggle to hear our inner voice, the more we can be said to be in a state of incongruence. According to this view, the various psychological problems we may experience are manifestations of the internalisation of conditions of worth.

In essence, what the theory is saying is that deep down each of us possesses an inner wisdom about how best to lead our lives. Each of us has a different best path to take in life, depending on our intrinsic characteristics, strengths, and interests. Unfortunately, few people ever find themselves on exactly the right path for them. We all know people who would make a brilliant teacher, a compassionate doctor, a talented carpenter, an inspired artist, but who for one reason or another never found their path in life to take them there. The brilliant teacher instead works as a sales director, the compassionate doctor is a civil servant, the carpenter is a journalist, and the inspired artist works in marketing and advertising. They might be good at what they do, but each feels that what they do is 'just not them'. Of course, it is not just about our employment, but this is the major way in which we come to express ourselves and our unique talents in our culture.

Thus, most of us realise only a fraction of our full potential. We grow up to develop an image of ourselves that we show to the world. We use psychological defences to stop us hearing the truth about this image. We do not want to hear evidence that we are not as clever, attractive, witty, handsome, or liked, as we tell ourselves. For this reason, we do not really get to know ourselves properly. We hide from knowing ourselves because the pain of self-knowledge is too great. In an unconditional and accepting social environment where we feel valued, however, we can begin to drop our defences and confront the truth about ourselves. That is the essence of client-centred therapy (CCT), which we will discuss in the next chapter.

Organismic valuing process

Although a mainstay of person-centred psychology (see Bozarth, 1998), the actualising tendency has been a controversial concept in mainstream psychology (see Ryan, 1995). Mainstream psychology has, as we have seen in Chapter 2, instead been more influenced by the legacy of psychoanalysis and the notion that human nature is rotten to the core (Seligman, 2003a).

As we have seen, the concept of the actualising tendency is somewhat revolutionary as it implies that people can trust themselves rather than so-called experts to know their own best directions in life (Joseph, 2003a). Thus, the task of the therapist is to help the person to listen, not to the therapist, but to their own inner voice of wisdom.

In talking about the inner voice of wisdom, Rogers (1964) used the term *organismic valuing process* (OVP). The OVP refers to people's innate ability to know what is important to them and what is essential for a fulfilling life. Rogers' view was that human organisms can be relied on through their physiological processes to know what they need from their environment and what is right for them for the self-actualisation of their potentialities. Similar ideas were expressed by Maslow:

> They listen to their own voices; they take responsibility; they are honest; and they work hard. They find out who they are and what they are, not only in terms of their mission in life, but also in terms of the way their feet hurt when they wear such and such a pair of shoes and whether they do or do not like eggplant . . . All this is what the real self means.
>
> (Maslow, 1993, p. 49)

Maslow describes how he would encourage his students to learn for themselves to listen to their own voices:

> I sometimes suggest to my students that when they are given a glass of wine and asked how they like it, they try a different way of responding. First, I suggest that they not look at the label on the bottle. Thus they will *not* use it to get any cue about whether or not they *should* like it. Next, I recommend that they close their eyes if possible and that they 'make a hush'. Now they are ready to look within themselves and try to shut out the noise of the world so that they may savor the wine on their tongues and look to the 'Supreme court' inside themselves.
>
> (Maslow, 1993, pp. 44–45)

This is an everyday exercise that all of us can try, and the point is to learn to apply this more generally in our lives, and to let the direction of our lives be guided by the 'supreme court' inside ourselves. One criticism that is sometimes made is that such an approach is a licence to let people do whatever they want and this would lead to destructive behaviour. This criticism is inevitably made by people with the fundamental assumption that human nature is destructive. From their point of view, it would, indeed, be chaotic if people were permitted to do whatever they wanted.

But it is not a licence to behave in whatever way we want, anyway. Of course, there must always be social constraints on how people behave to prevent harm. But the idea of letting people live their lives in accord with their own inner wisdom is an idea founded on the assumption that when people listen to that inner wisdom constructive behaviour and not destructive behaviour is the result. When people lead lives directed by their inner wisdom, they are, the theories of Rogers and Maslow suggest, self-directed, creative, autonomous, social, have an accurate view of themselves and other people, are willing to try and understand other people's points of view, and are open to new experiences. In Rogers' terminology, such people move toward becoming fully functioning. In Maslow's terminology, such people move towards self-actualisation.

The person-centred approach today

The person-centred approach remains highly influential in many settings. However, it has been less influential in mainstream psychology than in other healthcare disciplines, such as counselling and psychotherapy, where it remains an influential school of thought (Mearns & Thorne, 1999, 2000). Within psychology, however it has received much criticism. Although we would not dismiss these criticisms altogether, more often than not the criticisms are founded on a misperception of the theory itself. In part, this is due to Rogers himself leaving academia and, for the reasons discussed earlier, becoming less influential in mainstream psychology. The person-centred approach receives little coverage in today's psychology curriculum, and clinical psychologists in training may only have a few hours' exposure to the ideas and therapeutic approach of the person-centred model. As such, the only exposure that many of today's psychologists have had to the ideas of Rogers is through a page or two included in the 'perspectives on psychology' sections of introductory psychology textbooks. While not deliberately misrepresenting Rogers and his work, it is easy to see how only a superficial coverage can miss the profundity and complexity of Rogers' thinking, while presenting it inaccurately as an oversimplified approach that is deeply flawed. If this is all that a generation of psychologists have on which to base their understanding of Rogers and his work, it is no surprise that person-centred theory is misunderstood and misrepresented. Part of the misunderstanding and misrepresentation was fuelled because of the popularity of the approach during the 1970s, when the term person centred became appropriated by many whose work was superficial and poorly articulated, and would not have been considered person centred by the original developers of the approach.

Those within the person-centred movement have continued writing on the person-centred theory and practice, but their work has not been influential in mainstream psychology because of the misrepresentation we discussed earlier, and because it has tended to be published in books and periodicals, rather than in scientific journals. Person-centred practitioners and theorists have tended not to contribute significantly to the mainstream psychology's accepted research literature on theory and evidence-based practice, an agenda that has driven professional developments increasingly over the last few years. There are, of course, notable exceptions to this, but on balance, it is for these reasons that there is little mainstream psychological interest in the person-centred approach. But we must be cautious in how we interpret lack of evidence, since as already described, just because the evidence is not there, this does not automatically mean the ideas are not correct. In contrast, especially in relation to person-centred theory and client-centred therapy, it is much more the case that the research has simply not (yet) been done, and the questions have not (yet) been asked. However, with the advent of the positive psychology movement, times are changing. There is a growing recognition that there does indeed exist a vast resource of empirical research in the social and personality psychology tradition that is consistent with and supportive of the person-centred model (Patterson & Joseph, in press). The two movements of positive psychology and person-centred psychology are converging, and we explicate more fully later how they can both be used to inform and develop the other, especially in the context of positive therapy.

Positive psychology research

It is, we would argue, incorrect to criticise these early pioneers of humanistic psychology for not being scientific. In their day, they were at the forefront of scientific psychology. In particular, this is true of Carl Rogers. Criticisms of Rogers' approach have some-times been on the looseness of his language and the vagueness of his concepts, which critics have argued do not lend themselves to empirical testing. These criticisms may be justified from readings of his popular books, but certainly not from his peer reviewed scientific work. Client-centred therapy has a rich research history. Indeed, it is Rogers who is most often credited with introducing the field of psychotherapy research, recording his interviews on 78rpm records, which were then transcribed, and publishing the verbatim transcripts for research. A complete issue of the *Journal of Con-sulting Psychology* was devoted to the research in 1948 (see Farber, Brink, & Raskin, 1996). As well as pioneering psycho-therapy research, Rogers' theoretical statements about the neces-sary and sufficient conditions for personality change were certainly presented as empirically testable hypotheses (see Rogers, 1957, 1959). But, the perception among many is that it is an approach that is not well grounded in science. Although this is incorrect in the main (see Barrett-Lennard, 1998), it is true that there is little reason that the younger generation of psychologists should know otherwise, as we suggested earlier. Thus, we welcome positive psychology and the fact that it has begun to develop an empirical research base consistent within the person-centred approach.

What positive psychologists are able to bring to the ideas of earlier theorists such as Maslow and Rogers are the research techniques of current mainstream psychology (see Sheldon & Kasser, 2001). Forty years ago, when humanistic psychology was more mainstream than it is today, and these ideas were in popular currency, we simply did not have the methodological and statistical sophistication available to fully test the theories of Rogers and Maslow. At that time, psychological techniques were limited and the ideas of the behavioural psychologists were much more easily put to the test with the then primitive techniques.

Now we have sophisticated techniques that allow us to run statistical analyses in seconds that would have previously taken years, and the ability to test complicated multivariate models where we examine the summative and interactive effects of many different variables at once. The concept of the OVP is one such construct with revolutionary implications for the practice of psychology, but which has largely evaded scientific scrutiny. Although the OVP has been central to the theories of the humanistic writers like Rogers and Maslow, it has not attracted much empirical attention until recently within mainstream psychology (see Sheldon, Arndt, & Houser-Marko, 2003a; also developed more fully later).

However, even this statement about the lack of research is not strictly true. Certainly, there is now limited contemporary research under the name of person-centred theory, but social psychologists have continued working in related areas. There are aspects of person-centred theory that have gone on to be further developed in mainstream psychology by other theorists. Other theorists are in agreement with the basic premise of person-centred theory, i.e., that people have an innate tendency towards actualisation that can be either thwarted or facilitated by the social environment, and have developed a research tradition around these ideas.

So, although proponents of person-centred theory have not been as active in gathering empirical evidence as proponents of other therapeutic approaches, critics are wrong when they say that the person-centred approach lacks research evidence. There is a huge amount of evidence in support of person-centred theory but it is to be found in the journals of social and personality psychology, rather than the journals of counselling and clinical psychology. In particular, evidence is to be found in self-determination theory, which is one of the most influential theories in mainstream psychology in recent years, with striking similarities to person-centred theory, and which is supported by a substantial research effort (Patterson & Joseph, in press).

Rapprochement between positive psychology and the person-centred approach

Self-determination theory

Self-determination theory (SDT) (Deci & Ryan, 1985, 1991, 2000; Ryan & Deci, 2000) provides a similar meta-theoretical perspective to person-centred personality theory. SDT has three elements:

> The first is that human beings are inherently proactive, that they have the potential to act on and master both the inner forces (viz., their drives and emotions) and the external (i.e., environmental) forces they encounter, rather than being passively controlled by those forces . . .
> Second, human beings, as self-organizing systems, have an inherent tendency toward growth, development, and integrated functioning . . .
> The third important philosophical assumption is that, although activity and optimal development are inherent to the human organism, these do not happen automatically. For people to actualize their inherent nature and potentials – that is, to be optimally active and to develop effectively – they require nutrients from the social environment. To the extent that they are denied the necessary support and nourishment by chaotic, controlling, or rejecting environments, there will be negative consequences for their activity and development.
>
> (Deci & Vansteenkiste, 2004, pp. 23–24)

Although SDT theorists trace the different lineage of their work to Harlow (1953) and White (1959), rather than directly to Rogers (1959), as will be evident from the previous chapter these are the same meta-theoretical elements that also constitute Rogers' person-centred personality theory (Rogers, 1959). At the meta-theoretical level, SDT and person-centred theory are synonymous (Patterson & Joseph, in press). This is an exciting convergence of ideas from these two traditions of psychological thought.

Mainstream psychological practice, however, adopts the opposite position to these three elements with their agenda of therapist expertise and implicit assumption that motivation for development needs to be externally imposed on the person. As we have argued throughout this book, and elsewhere (Linley & Joseph, 2004c), these meta-theoretical elements promise to provide the foundation stone for positive psychology, and, we hope, eventually for psychology as a whole. Similarly, Deci and Vansteenkiste (2004) write:

> Although positive psychology researchers are working to identify factors that enhance individuals' capacities, development, and well-being, only a few . . . fully embrace and utilize this critical meta-theoretical assumption for grounding their research or building their theoretical perspectives.
> (Deci & Vansteenkiste, 2004, p. 24)

Thus, we are beginning to see how there is indeed a massive amount of contemporary positive social psychological theory and research in support of person-centred theory and the concept of intrinsic motivation, and for the role of the social environment.

Research evidence

Positive psychologists such as Deci and Vansteenkiste (2004) and Ryan (1995) are in agreement that the organismic valuing process is either supported or undermined by the social environment. However, whereas Rogers emphasised the universal need people have for unconditional positive regard from the social environment, SDT posits thus three basic psychological needs – autonomy, competence, and relatedness – and theorises that fulfilment of these needs is essential for growth. The need for autonomy concerns the need to be able to act through choice and volition. The need for competence concerns the need to be effective in dealing with the environment. The need for relatedness concerns the need to connect with others.

Similarly to the concept of unconditional positive regard, these are not conceptualised as learned needs, but as an inherent aspect of human nature that can be seen across gender, across time, and across culture (Chirkov, Ryan, Kim, & Kaplan, 2003). Deci and Vansteenkiste (2004) and Ryan (1995) have emphasised how the social environment must provide the nutrients to provide for individuals' needs for autonomy, relatedness, and competence. People are intrinsically motivated to move towards social environments that provide these needs.

SDT therefore defines the nutrients that the social environment must provide for intrinsic motivation to take place. Deci and Ryan (2000) agree that the social environment does not always meet these needs, and that when these needs are not met development is thwarted leading to ill-being, and alienation. Thus, whereas Rogers talked generally about condition of worth – those ways of behaving that we have learned from experience that make us acceptable to others – that thwart the actualising tendency, Deci and Ryan have provided a broadly similar account of the same processes. SDT and person-centred theory obviously share much common ground and we are left with some questions for future research and theoretical discussion. Theoretically, it is not clear from the writings of Deci and Ryan whether an unconditionally and positively regarding social environment as posited by Rogers (1957, 1959) sufficiently provides the organism with the nutrients to develop autonomy, competence, and relatedness. Our reading of Rogers (1959) suggests that the answer be yes. In Rogers' (1959) definition of the actualising tendency, the organism is intrinsically motivated toward autonomy, competence, and relatedness.

Examination of existing evidence suggests that research supporting SDT is equally supportive of person-centred theory, and humanistic theories more generally (Sheldon, Joiner, Pettit, & Williams, 2003b). Deci and Ryan's conceptualisation of need satisfactions is not that different from that of unconditional positive regard. For example, Deci and Ryan, and their colleagues have used self-report questionnaires to measure the concept of needs satisfaction. In one study by La Guardia, Ryan, Couchman, and Deci (2000) looking at parental influence, when we examine sample items from that used to measure autonomy (e.g., *my mother allows me to decide things for myself*), competence (e.g., *my mother puts time and energy into helping me*), and relatedness (e.g., *my mother accepts me and likes me as I am*), we can see very clearly that these items could equally well be conceptualised as measuring the broader concept of unconditional positive regard: unconditionality (e.g., *my mother allows me to decide things for myself*), and positive regard (e.g., *my mother accepts me and likes me as I am*). The difference between unconditional positive regard and needs satisfaction might therefore simply be terminological, an issue that requires further theoretical and empirical clarification.

One of the main findings in SDT research, replicated many times, and confirmed in meta-analysis, is that people are less likely to engage in activities that they find interesting when the rewards for that activity are extrinsic (e.g., money) (Deci, Koestner, & Ryan, 1999). But, when the social environment supports autonomy, for example through increased choice, then intrinsic motivation is enhanced (Reeve, Nix, & Hamm, 2003).

SDT makes the case, similar to Rogers (1959), that intrinsic motivation is necessarily autonomous, but this is not the case with extrinsic motivations. Ryan (1995) distinguished between external regulation (i.e., doing something out of fear of punishment), introjected regulation (i.e., doing something to avoid feeling guilty), identified regulation (i.e., doing something because the values are endorsed), and integrated regulation (i.e., where the person has integrated the identification with the self). In Rogers' (1959) person-centred personality theory, conditions of worth are viewed developmentally: beginning as externally regulated, as when a child does something to avoid punishment, becoming introjected, and finally identified and integrated. Through the process of therapy, as we shall see in the next chapter, this process is put into reverse.

What we wanted to show was that our approach to positive therapy and its grounding in person-centred personality theory is part of a wider movement in positive psychology towards the adoption of this meta-theoretical perspective. Research evidence is supportive. We are also beginning to see research that is supportive of the concept of the OVP. In a series of three studies, for example, Sheldon et al. (2003a) examined how people changed their mind over time about what goals and values to pursue. Their rationale was that evidence for the existence of an OVP would be demonstrated by people's tendency to move toward well-being related outcomes, such as those to do with intrinsic goals as opposed to extrinsic goals. Their results provide evidence that participants evidenced relatively greater ratings shifts towards goals that are more likely to be beneficial to their well-being.

Other work into the longitudinal effects of self-concordant goal selection shows that those with more self-concordant goals (i.e., those who pursue goals for intrinsic rather than extrinsic reasons) put more sustained effort into those goals, which enables them to better attain those goals. Goal attainment in turn is associated with stronger feelings of autonomy, competence, and relatedness, which in turn lead to greater well-being (Sheldon & Elliot, 1999). The evidence suggests that people grow when there is contact with the OVP. Other work shows that teenagers with mothers who are high in warmth and democratic parenting are more likely to hold intrinsic values and goals (Kasser, Ryan, Zax, & Sameroff, 1995; Williams, Cox, Hedberg, & Deci, 2000).

There remains much further research work to be conducted into the existence of an OVP. However, we believe that the emerging positive psychology research in this area suggests that the organismic valuing process might be set centre stage as the fundamental pillar of positive therapy. This approach is very much consistent with the findings from positive psychology research traditions. For example, the positive influence on well-being created by intrinsic aspirations (Carver & Baird, 1998; Chan & Joseph, 2000; Kasser, 2004; Kasser & Ryan, 1993, 1996), intrinsic motivation (Deci & Ryan, 1985, 1991, 2000; Ryan & Deci, 2000), intrinsic yearning to use one's signature strengths (Peterson & Seligman, 2003), and the concept of flow (Csikszentmihalyi, 1990, 1997), have all been extensively documented. Thus, when we examine this weight of theory and evidence we see a real rapprochement between positive psychology and the person-centred approach. We concur with Sheldon and Elliot (1999) who wrote:

[A]long with Rogers (1961), we believe that individuals have innate developmental trends and propensities that may be given voice by an organismic valueing process occurring within them. The voice can be very difficult to hear, but the current research suggests that the ability to hear it is of crucial importance for the pursuit of happiness.
(Sheldon & Elliot, 1999, p. 495)

Criticisms of the person-centred approach

Thus, our view is that the person-centred approach offers a genuinely positive psychological perspective. How is it then that the person-centred approach has been so marginalised and besieged in psychology? In large part, critics of the person-centred approach have simply misunderstood the theory. Many of the criticisms are simply not valid when one is able properly to understand and appreciate the depth and complexity of person-centred personality theory, rather than the 'strawman' of this theory that is often found in introductory texts.

As we have seen already, the first major criticism is that the person-centred approach is a licence to let people do whatever they want, which would result in chaos. But this is to misunderstand the idea, which is to be expected when one understands that the critics inevitably have contrasting fundamental assumptions. From their point of view, if people were to listen to their inner voice rather than external sources of control, there would indeed be chaos as the inner voice would be that of conflicting destructive impulses. Rather, person-centred theory emphasises the importance of an unconditionally accepting social environment characterised by empathy and genuineness. This is not the same thing as suggesting that therapists do nothing. Quite the opposite, client-centred therapy is an active therapy, providing acceptance, empathy, and authenticity is hard work. But when a person perceives themselves to be accepted, valued, and understood, there is growth in a socially constructive direction. But as Sheldon and Elliot (1999) note, the inner voice is not easy to hear and takes some consider-able experience to do so.

Thus, the theory recognises that personal growth is a difficult process and that people can behave in destructive ways. There is no denial in person-centred theory of the need for social control, it is just not the task of the person-centred therapist to provide it. Person-centred psychologists do not deny the cruelty and suffering in the world, but they do not see counselling and psychotherapy as an agent for the provision of this social control. Social control is needed and can be implemented by police, prisons, and arguably those mental health professionals working from other meta-theoretical assumptions to the person-centred philosophy, who have either stepped willingly into the role of agents of social control, or who have unknowingly confused the task of personal transformation with that of social control – a point that we will return to in Chapter 8.

A second criticism of Rogers' ideas is to view his emphasis on the actualising tendency as evidence of his 'Pollyanna' theorising. If humans do have an innate ability to know what is important to them and what is essential for a fulfilling life, how is it that so many are distressed and dysfunctional? But again this is to mis-understand the concept of the actualising tendency and the OVP as it is developed in the person-centred theory proposed by Rogers, and similarly with SDT. As we shall show later, person-centred theory, and SDT, do not suggest that people are always social and constructive. The theory also provides a sophisticated account of psychopathology and why it is that people often behave in destructive ways (Wilkins, 2005a). The actualising tendency becomes thwarted and usurped so that the person self-actualises in a destructive and dysfunctional way.

It is understandable that practitioners of other approaches, when they misunderstand the theory as suggesting that people are always good, are critical. Given the horrors of the last century, and the fact that the world is full of people causing each other harm and distress, surely it is just naïve, they say, to think that people are intrinsically motivated toward growth, development, positive and constructive functioning. But this criticism is to misunderstand person-centred theory. It is, of course, naïve to think that people *always behave* in a positive and constructive way, but person-centred personality theory just does not say that they do. Rather, what it says is that at core people have one motivational force toward growth and development, the *actualising tendency*, and this force leads us to be *intrinsically motivated toward* positive and constructive functioning that is consistent with the needs of the person as an organism. But, under unfavourable social–environmental conditions the actualising tendency becomes usurped by extrinsic forces so that the direction of self-actualisation becomes *incongruent* with the organismic needs manifest in the actualising tendency leading instead to growth and development that is negative and destructive, and working at cross-purposes with the intrinsic motivation toward positive and constructive functioning (Ford, 1991).

Conclusion

We began this chapter by asking the question how should we decide on our artistry as therapists? If we assume the existence of the OVP, then our task as therapists is to facilitate the OVP and to assist the client in hearing their own inner voice. How do we go about helping people to hear the inner voice of wisdom within themselves? Our view at present is that what positive psychology tells us about personality processes leads us to formulate a framework for therapy that is largely consistent with the person-centred approaches to therapy. The critical point here is that the locus of responsibility for the direction of the therapy is with the client, rather than with the therapist. It is self-evident that if the task of therapy is to help people to hear their own inner voice more clearly, then it is important that the voice of the therapist does not drown out the voice of the client. This is not to say that the therapist is silent, on the contrary, the therapist should be an active agent in the process of facilitating the client to listen to him or herself better.

We shall go on to describe this in more detail in Chapter 4. For the moment, however, what we want to emphasise is how revolutionary the implications of the person-centred approach are. The world is full of individuals and organisations that purport to know better than we do ourselves about how we should choose to live our lives, and what we should believe. The person-centred approach rejects this, and says instead that each of us is our own best expert on ourselves. In terms of therapeutic practice, it is the therapist's trust in the person's actualising tendency that makes the person-centred approach, and those other humanistic and positive therapy approaches that adopt this stance, so radically different from other therapeutic approaches. But psychologists who have not appreciated the profound significance of this view, that it is the client and not the therapist who knows best what direction to go in, often misunderstand client-centred psychotherapy. A common criticism of the client-centred approach is that if people knew best what direction to go in, then they would not need to seek help from a therapist. But this is to misunderstand the nature of the actualising tendency as described by Rogers. It is not easy to hear one's inner voice of wisdom, but the task is to help our clients to do just this. Positive psychologists, as we have seen, are reexamining the concept of the actualising tendency, and the available evidence is consistent with the existence of an organismic valuing process that reliably guides us toward knowing our own best directions in life, and the steps that we should take to achieve our own optimal health and well-being.

Chapter 4

Client-centred therapy and positive therapies

In Chapter 3, we examined in detail person-centred personality theory and some of the supporting evidence from positive psychology, concluding that person-centred theory provides us with a framework for understanding well-being. Person-centred theory, in turn, underlies the practice of client-centred therapy. In turning to consider therapy practice, we think it might first of all be helpful if we first describe in some detail what client-centred therapy looks like and also how it relates to some current positive psychology constructs. The crux of client-centred therapy, and its defining feature, is the therapist's trust in the client's own actualising tendency and that given the right social environmental conditions, self-actualisation will be congruent with the actualising tendency. Thus, what the therapist tries to do is to provide the right social environmental conditions. Rogers (1957) described six conditions that he held were necessary and sufficient for positive therapeutic change. It is worth noting that Rogers believed these conditions to underlie *any* therapeutic personality change, and thus believed that they must be in operation in any successful therapy. They were not considered to be restricted solely to client-centred therapy, which is unfortunately a common misconception, and leads to the unfounded criticism of 'well, we do that already', when the six conditions are presented to a therapist from another therapeutic perspective. This is a point to which we return later.

Six necessary and sufficient conditions

In terms of what the client-centred therapist actually does to facilitate the client in hearing their own inner voice, Rogers (1957) stated that there were six necessary and sufficient conditions,

Table 4.1 Necessary and sufficient conditions of constructive
personality change

1	Two persons are in psychological contact
2	The first, whom we shall call the client, is in a state of incongruence, being vulnerable or anxious
3	The second person, whom we shall call the therapist, is congruent or integrated in the relationship
4	The therapist experiences unconditional positive regard for the client
5	The therapist experiences an empathic understanding of the client's internal frame of reference and endeavours to communicate this experience to the client
6	The communication to the client of the therapist's empathic understanding and unconditional positive regard is to a minimal degree achieved

Source: Rogers, 1957, p. 96

which, when present, provided the social environment that facilitated the OVP (see Table 4.1).

Condition 1 is referring to a precondition that, if not met, would mean that the following five conditions were redundant. What Rogers means by *psychological contact* is whether or not the two people are aware of each other, and that the behaviour of one impacts on the other. So, for example, if someone were in a catatonic state, it would be difficult to judge whether there was psychological contact.

In the second condition, *incongruence* is explained as consisting of an incompatibility between underlying feelings and awareness of those feelings, or an incompatibility between awareness of feelings and the expression of feelings. For example, someone who appears anxious to an observer but has no awareness themselves of feeling anxious would be said to be incongruent in terms of their underlying feelings and their awareness of those feelings. Someone who is aware of their anxiety but says that they are feeling relaxed would be said to be incongruent between awareness and expression.

In the third condition, the therapist is congruent, that is to say, he or she is aware of their inner experience, e.g., feelings of anger, sadness, and is able to express this openly and honestly if thought to be appropriate.

In the fourth condition, the therapist is able to provide *unconditional positive regard*, that is to say, he or she is able to accept the client without imposing conditions of worth on the client.

In the fifth condition, the therapist has *empathic understanding*; that is to say, he or she is able to sense what the client's experience must feel like.

Finally, in the sixth condition, the client perceives the therapist's empathy and unconditional acceptance. Rogers believed that if these six conditions were in existence then constructive personality change would occur, but only if all six were present, and the more that they were present the more marked would be the constructive personality change of the client.

Rogers was saying that all psychotherapies are effective insofar as the necessary and sufficient conditions are present. The necessary and sufficient conditions were an integrative statement and not a description of client-centred psychotherapy per se. Certainly, the necessary and sufficient conditions outlined by Rogers (1957) describe the attitudinal qualities of the client-centred psychotherapist, their congruence, empathy, and unconditional positive regard. Conditions 3, 4, and 5 are referred to as the *core conditions* and describe the practice of the client-centred therapist – they endeavour to be congruent, empathic, and to experience unconditional positive regard for their client. Within the client-centred movement, there has been a tremendous amount of further writing on the necessary and sufficient conditions (see e.g., Bozarth & Wilkins, 2001; Haugh & Merry, 2001; Wyatt, 2001; Wyatt & Sanders, 2001), but it is not our intention to go into the detail on this literature here, but rather to illustrate the main ideas and to show how these ideas are still relevant today to contemporary positive psychologists.

This 1957 paper of Rogers describing the six conditions is one of the most well-known of all of his papers, and for many outside the client-centred movement it is often seen as the essence of client-centred therapy. But is this not what all therapist do anyway? We don't think so. As Brazier put it:

> When people read about Rogers' ideas, it is not uncommon for them to think initially that there is nothing very remarkable about them. Do we not all believe in the importance of people being empathic to one another? What is so remarkable about that? What is remarkable is that Rogers actually meant it. And in carrying through what are essentially a very simple set of ideas whose rightness seems self-evident, he offers a challenge to the foundations of most of what modern life consists of.
>
> (Brazier, 1993, p. 8)

Many critics of the client-centred approach confuse these core conditions with client-centred therapy. But as we have seen, the fundamental idea of client-centred therapy is that these core attitudinal qualities are the social environment that foster what Rogers called the actualising tendency. It is this aspect of theory that makes sense of the core conditions theoretically. We saw this in the previous chapter, that when the social environment is characterised by unconditional positive regard the person is more able to actualise in the direction of their intrinsic motivational force toward autonomy, competence, and relatedness, and thus to become more fully functioning. The crux of client-centred therapy is the provision, by the therapist, to the client, of an unconditionally accepting social environment. In such an environment, where a person does not feel judged or evaluated, they no longer feel the need to defend themselves, and can begin the process of listening to themselves, and their own inner voice of wisdom, the organismic valuing process.

Thus, conditions 3, 4, and 5 are referred to as the core conditions and describe the practice of the client-centred therapist – they endeavour to be congruent, empathic, and to experience unconditional positive regard for their client, in the belief that by doing so it helps to release the intrinsic motivation of the person toward autonomy, relatedness, and competence, and away from the denial and defence that characterise psychopathology.

However, eclectic or integrative therapists often describe themselves as using client-centred therapy because they endeavour to be empathic, congruent, and unconditionally regarding, but without their belief in the clients actualising tendency it is simply incorrect to call what they do as client centred. It is the belief in the actualising tendency that provides the theoretical rationale for the therapeutic provision of an unconditionally accepting attitude, empathy, and congruence. In an attempt to explain this using the analogy of psychoanalysis:

> It is the belief in the actualising tendency that sets client-centred psychotherapy apart from other therapy traditions. It might be said that the actualising tendency is to client-centred psychotherapy what the unconscious is to psychoanalysis. It would be nonsense for a therapist to claim to practise psychoanalysis just because they used free association techniques if they did not also believe that there were unconscious forces

shaping behaviour. Similarly, it would be nonsense for therapists to claim to practise client-centred psychotherapy just because they endeavour to accept their client unconditionally if they do not hold in the first place that there is an actualising tendency.

(Joseph, 2003a, p. 305)

Also, it is the *combination* of the six conditions that is important. It is no use the therapist only having an unconditionally accepting attitude; the client must experience the therapist's attitude as being unconditionally accepting. This is where empathy and congruence come in, since these are the vehicles for the transmission of unconditional positive regard (Bozarth, 1998). Congruence and empathy are central to practice because the best vantage point for understanding behaviour is from the internal frame of reference of the individual themselves. Rogers (1951) argued that the only way we could understand another person's behaviour was to see the world through their eyes. Then, even the most seemingly bizarre behaviour would make meaningful sense.

Thus, the crux of client-centred therapy is not the provision of the core conditions per se that characterise client-centred therapy, but the therapist's meta-theoretical assumption that people are intrinsically motivated towards constructive and optimal functioning and that under the right social environmental conditions this force is released:

> Client-centered therapists make no assumptions about what people need or how they should be free. They do not attempt to promote self-acceptance, self-direction, positive growth, self-actualization, congruence between real or perceived selves, a particular vision of reality, or anything . . . *Client-centered therapy is the practice of simply respecting the right to self-determination of others.*
>
> (Grant, 2004, p. 158)

It is that respect for the self-determination of others that underpins the unconditional attitude of the therapist and the principled stance of non-directivity, which is the distinguishing feature of the approach (see Levitt, 2005b). As Brodley (2005b) wrote:

> The non-directive attitude is psychologically profound; it is not a technique. Early in a therapist's development it may be

superficial and prescriptive – 'Don't do this' or 'Don't do that'. But with time, self-examination and therapy experience, it becomes an aspect of the therapist's character. It represents a feeling of profound respect for the constructive potential in persons and great sensitivity to their vulnerability.

(p. 3)

Evidence base

A central question for any audience of psychologists is inevitably whether or not client-centred psychotherapy is an effective way of helping people. Early research throughout the 1960s provided evidence consistent with Rogers' hypothesis of the necessary and sufficient conditions (Truax & Mitchell, 1971; see Barrett-Lennard, 1998). However, over the next two decades the research tradition in client-centred psychotherapy dwindled, in large part because the new generation of research active psychologists tended to be interested in the new cognitive approach to psychotherapy, and client-centred psychotherapy became increasingly a marginalised approach within mainstream psychology (for the reasons we have already described in Chapter 3). As a consequence, the question of whether the six conditions posited by Rogers are necessary and sufficient remains largely unanswered, with different researchers interpreting the available data very differently indeed. This really is remarkable, since people have tended to dismiss the client-centred approach without ever giving it proper consideration, whereas cognitive-behavioural approaches have found wide acceptance largely because they readily lend themselves easily to the requirements of scientific research. However, as we have seen, when client-centred therapy and cognitive-behavioural therapy were compared as treatments for depression, both approaches were found to be equally effective (King et al., 2000). Notwithstanding this, researchers from traditions other than the client-centred one have tended to interpret the evidence to suggest that the conditions might be necessary, but that they are not sufficient. Consequently, there is seen to be a need by therapists from other traditions to further intervene in some way, for example, using various cognitive or behavioural techniques.

However, client-centred therapists have interpreted the same data to suggest that the conditions might not be necessary, but that they are sufficient. It is thought that personal development and growth can also come about through a variety of vehicles of change, from religious conversions to traumatic experiences, and so the conditions might not be necessary, but when they are present they are sufficient (see Bozarth, 1998, for a review). There is, therefore, no need for further intervention.

But whether or not the conditions are necessary or sufficient, most therapists from whatever orientation would agree that these relationship factors are at least important contributory factors to therapeutic personality change. The evidence for the role of the relationship is overwhelming (see Bozarth & Motomasa, 2005; Wampold, 2001). In a study of the treatment of depression, across all therapies, Krupnick et al. (1996) found that the relationship contributed one-fifth of the outcome variance, a finding that is consistent across therapies (Lambert, 1992), and which is second only to the resources of the client themselves in predicting a successful therapeutic outcome (Duncan & Miller, 2000; Hubble & Miller, 2004; Wampold, 2001).

There is now considerable scope for future process-oriented research to assess the experience of therapeutic conditions and how they relate to subsequent outcome. Process research is important if we are to understand more about how psychotherapy works. The client-centred approach has been criticised for not lending itself to research. But this is not the case, and researchers in the past have developed psychometric tools based on person-centred theory that can be used to test aspects of personal-centred theory. For example, the Barrett-Lennard relationship inventory (BLRI) (Barrett-Lennard, 1986) can be used to assess perceptions of empathy, congruence, and unconditional positive regard from the client's perspective, and how these perceptions relate to later outcome (see Table 4.2 for example items).

However, on a day-to-day basis, therapists are often more concerned with simply whether or not the therapy is effective. Recent outcome research using randomised-controlled trials has shown that client-centred psychotherapy was more effective than routine care from general practitioners for depression (Friedli, King, Lloyd, & Horder, 1997). More recently, client-centred psychotherapy has also been shown to be as effective as cognitive-behavioural treatments in the alleviation of depression. As noted earlier, King et al. (2000) found no difference between cognitive-behavioural therapy offered by clinical psychologists and client-centred psychotherapy offered by person-centred counsellors in the

Table 4.2 Example items from the BLRI

- My therapist wants to understand how I see things
- My therapist nearly always knows exactly what I mean
- I feel that my therapist is real and genuine with me
- My therapist is friendly and warm with me
- I feel that my therapist really values me
- My therapist is openly himself/herself in our relationship

treatment of depression. This again very much raises the question of what are the key factors in successful therapeutic outcome, and clearly suggest that there is much more going on than 'just' the therapeutic technique. Indeed, recent advances point fundamentally to the role of the client in successful therapeutic outcome, suggesting that as much as 40–87 percent of outcome variance may be attributable to client factors alone, followed by relationship factors, with therapeutic orientation coming a distant third place (Bozarth & Motomasa, 2005; Duncan & Miller, 2000; Hubble & Miller, 2004; Wampold, 2001). Clearly, the client seems to have been unduly forgotten in psychotherapy research, and client-centred approaches could do much to reintroduce a consideration of the impact of the client into scientific research protocols (Hubble & Miller, 2004; Joseph & Linley, 2004, 2005).

Client-centred therapy and positive psychology

The terminology of Rogers' (1957, 1959) theory will be familiar to psychologists, few of whom will not have heard the terms unconditional positive regard, empathy, and congruence. However, it is perhaps the case that these terms are so familiar that the depth of the theory is often overlooked, and is mistaken for a much more superficial approach than it truly is. Sometimes we think we understand something so well already that it is hard to see it differently. We suspect that something of this nature occurs when many psychologists are introduced to client-centred therapy. We have talked with many very senior clinical psychologists who simply do not understand the principle of client-centred therapy, and who think it is a naïve and superficial approach. This, in itself, betrays only a naïve and superficial understanding of the principles of client-centred therapy.

At core, as we have seen, is the idea that all therapists operate on the basis of deep-seated personal world views, or fundamental assumptions, that they bring into the consulting room, and which influence their way of being with another person. However, we have also heard senior consultant clinical psychologists argue that they do not hold any underlying fundamental assumptions, but that as scientist–practitioners, they are able to draw on different theories as appropriate in the treatment of their clients. As we have seen, though, it simply does not make sense to believe one day that people are their own best experts and the next day to believe otherwise, without seeming confused and contradictory in your way of being with your clients.

It is understandable that clinicians trained in the therapist-as-expert model, who are not aware of any alternative, can experience themselves as moving around eclectically between different therapeutic approaches, one day offering behavioural intervention, the next cognitive, and yet the next psychodynamic, without realising that, at core, what they are doing each day is essentially the same, i.e., offering themselves as the expert on the other person, the client.

However, we are encouraged by the new generation of psychologists who are drawn to the ideas of positive psychology. As the positive psychological perspective informs the thinking of this new generation, we are confident that the prejudices that undermine client-centred therapy will be overcome, and the approach will be able to be evaluated more fairly on its merits. We believe that the ideas of person-centred psychology are simply too good to keep down, and that ultimately client-centred therapy will be more widely recognised and respected for what it offers. Certainly, it might not be the answer to all human ills, but the philosophical stance of respecting other people's right to self-determination is an important one that we ought not to disregard on the basis of ethics alone. However, we also recognise and acknowledge that Rogers' language can now seem dated, and as such, we have attempted to reframe the core conditions of client-centred therapy within current more mainstream terminology.

Relating the 1957 statement of Rogers, describing the six necessary and sufficient conditions of personality change, to current terminology, we would describe client-centred therapy as a profound experiential approach founded on the *emotional intelligence* of the therapist.

Emotional intelligence

The basis of the client-centred therapeutic approach is condition 3, the therapist's congruence. Congruence refers to the person's awareness of their underlying thoughts and feelings, and their ability to express these thoughts and feelings appropriately in the context (Bozarth, 1998; Wyatt, 2001). That is to say, there is congruence between the internal cognitive and emotional states of the person, their conscious awareness of those states, and their ability to articulate the expression of those states.

Congruence, when combined with condition 5, empathic understanding, would involve all four facets of emotional intelligence as discussed by Salovey, Caruso, and Mayer (2004; Salovey, Mayer, & Caruso, 2002). The congruent therapist who has an empathic understanding of the client's frame of reference is:

1   perceptive of how the client is feeling
2   perceptive of how they themselves are feeling
3   able to manage their own emotions and to use their own emotions creatively in the service of the therapeutic relationship
4   able to understand emotions and to label them appropriately.

What this means in practice is that the client-centred therapist is someone who has a deep understanding of themselves and is able to be present in an authentic way with the client. The therapist strives to understand the client's world from the client's perspective, and they are accepting of the client's directions in life without imposing their own agenda, that is to say, the self-determination of the client is paramount.

Self-determination

This last point, being accepting of the client's directions without imposing one's own, is as we have seen already, the crux of client-centred therapy (i.e., condition 4) and is communicated through the therapist's congruence and empathy (see Bozarth, 1998). It is fundamental to the client-centred therapist, because of his or her trust in the actualising tendency as the one central source of human motivation, that they do not intervene, and have no intention of intervening. As Bozarth (1998) put it:

The therapist goes with the client, goes at the client's pace, goes with the client in his/her own ways of thinking, of experiencing, or processing. The therapist cannot be up to other things, have other intentions without violating the essence of person-centred therapy. To be up to other things – whatever they might be – is a 'yes, but' reaction to the essence of the approach. It must mean that when the therapist has intentions of treatment plans, of treatment goals, of interventive strategies to get the client somewhere or for the client to do a certain thing, the therapist violates the essence of person-centred therapy.

(Bozarth, 1998, pp. 11–12)

Authentic relationship

What we want to emphasise most of all is how client-centred therapy allows for tremendous variety and spontaneity in ways of working. No two client-centred therapists will be the same, as it is an approach to therapy that is founded on the therapists' emotional intelligence. Essentially, the idea is that within an authentic and emotionally literate relationship, people are able to drop their defences and get to know themselves better, and feel free to make new choices in life. Person-centred theory says that, in such relationships, people move to make new and wiser choices for themselves by listening more to their organismic valuing process, the inner voice of wisdom within us all.

Client-centred therapy is about the authentic quality of the relationship between the therapist and client. Decades of therapy research suggest that Rogers' (1957) statement was close to the mark in pointing to the central importance of the therapeutic relationship (see Martin, Garske, & Davis, 2000; Wampold, 2001). What we do know, with as much certainty as it is possible to have, and as we discussed earlier, is that successful therapy is not due to particular therapeutic techniques, levels of training, or the use of diagnosis.

The recent findings of the American Psychological Association Division 29 Task Force on empirically supported therapy relationships (Norcross, 2001) show that it is the therapeutic relationship and the client's own inner resources that are important. This is a conclusion now reached by many researchers (e.g., Bozarth, 1998; Bozarth & Motomasa, 2005; Duncan & Miller, 2000;

Hubble & Miller, 2004; Martin et al., 2000; Wampold, 2001) and which can be taken as evidence for the person-centred approach (Cornelius-White, 2002). Further, analyses of the factors that contribute to the development of a positive working alliance (i.e., effective therapeutic relationship) also accord with the central tenets of client-centred therapy. For example, therapists' personal qualities of being flexible, honest, respectful, trustworthy, confident, warm, interested, and open have been shown to contribute positively to a better working alliance. Therapist techniques of exploration, reflection, noting past therapy success, accurate interpretation, facilitating expression of affect, and attending to the client's experience also contribute positively to the alliance (see Ackerman & Hilsenroth, 2003).

The actualising tendency as fundamental

As we have seen it is the belief in the actualising tendency that sets client-centred counselling and psychotherapy apart from other therapy traditions (Bozarth, 1998; Joseph, 2003a). As we have seen already, it would be nonsense for therapists to claim to practise client-centred therapy just because they endeavour to be empathic, congruent, and unconditionally accepting of their client, if they do not hold in the first place that there is an actualising tendency. These core attitudinal qualities of the therapist only make sense in relation to the meta-theoretical perspective of person-centred theory. This is what is so often misunderstood by therapists who claim to be eclectic. Endeavouring to be empathic, congruent, and unconditionally accepting is not in itself client-centred therapy: one must also hold and respect that the actualising tendency is the client's source of motivation.

Belief in the actualising tendency has profound implications for practice. A therapist endeavouring to hold the conditions of empathy, congruence, and unconditional positive regard, but who is not trusting in this one central source of energy in the human organism – the actualising tendency – is not practising client-centred therapy. It is the client-centred psychotherapist's trust in the actualising tendency that makes the approach so revolutionary (Bozarth, 1998). Most other therapeutic approaches take the stance that the therapist is the expert who intervenes in some way to help the client resolve their problem.

Rogers' view was that given the right social environmental conditions, clients will be able to find their own directions, and that these directions will always be constructive, and toward becoming more fully functioning. This is the crux of person-centred approach. Therapists who take on the role of expert thus run the risk that they inadvertently serve to thwart the actualising tendency of their client, and consequently impede their client in becoming more able to find their own directions. We are therefore cautious in introducing the concept of the positive therapies as a broad umbrella to emphasise that person-centred theory is the central stem. In talking about the range of therapies that may fall under the umbrella of the positive therapies, we emphasise that the defining features of positive therapy are, first of all, that the client is their own best expert – not the therapist – and, second, that therapy is about the relationship – not the technique.

The family of person-centred therapies

Although the approach to classical client-centred therapy practised today remains very much that developed by Rogers, client-centred psychotherapy is not an approach stranded in the 1950s and 1960s. There has been much theoretical and practical development in the world of client-centred psychotherapy over recent years (see e.g., Joseph & Worsley, 2005a; Levitt, 2005b; Mearns & Thorne, 2000; Sanders, 2004; Thorne & Lambers, 1998; Warner, 2005; Worsley, 2001).

As well as developments within what might be described as the classical approach to client-centred psychotherapy, others have proposed what they see as ways of working therapeutically that integrate other ideas. For example, Rennie (1998) has developed what he sees as a reflexive and more experiential way of working that draws on existential and interpersonal therapy, and his extensive qualitative research into the clients' subjective experiences (Rennie, 1996).

Of practical interest have been the attempts to find ways of working within the client-centred framework with people whose psychological contact is at a very minimum level, and who may therefore struggle to meet the first condition, that of psychological contact. Prouty (1990) has developed an approach called pre-therapy, which involves reflecting back to the client the counsellor's awareness of the client's external world and communication with others. Pre-therapy aims to help the client develop psychological contact in order that they can then enter more conventional therapy. Pre-therapy approaches have been used with some success in helping people suffering from problems of psychosis (Prouty, Van Werde, & Portner, 2002; Van Werde, 1998, 2005).

Other approaches that are sometimes considered as part of the family of person-centred approaches are the experiential focusing approach (Gendlin, 1996), and the process-experiential approach (Greenberg, Rice, & Elliott, 1993). Although these approaches hold that the process of therapy can be helped along with the use of more directive methods than are associated with more traditional client-centred psychotherapy, they maintain the view that it is the client's own inner process that will lead them to finding solutions to their problems. This is the crux of what it means to be client centred, and as we enter the new century, the view that it is the client and not the therapist who knows best what direction to take is again a powerful and revolutionary idea (see also Duncan & Miller, 2000; Hubble & Miller, 2004).

Thus, the idea of the client as expert can be interpreted in various ways in practice, ranging from the classical client-centred approach to therapy (Merry, 2004), with its principled role of going with the client, at the client's pace, through to more existential (Cooper, 2004, 2005), experiential (Baker, 2004), and process-directed approaches in which the therapist may introduce various exercises into the sessions (Worsley, 2001, 2004; and see Chapter 5). Later we will consider some of the other broad meta-approaches that we think resonate with the general positive therapy orientation that we have been describing. Namely, they hold that the client is their own best expert, they adopt a non-medical model viewpoint, and they provide an integrative view of negative and positive human experience. Specifically here, we briefly consider Eastern approaches to therapy, and existential approaches to therapy. In Chapter 5, we will extend this consideration to take more account of process-oriented therapies that might be considered under the positive therapy umbrella.

Positive therapies

Eastern approaches

Although it is not often made explicit, client-centred therapies have much in common with therapeutic approaches derived from

Eastern traditions. The relation between the client-centred approach and the tradition of Zen is explored by Brazier (1995) who discusses how Zen is a form of therapy:

> The challenge which Zen poses us is to reach deeply into the experience of being alive to find something authentic . . . Zen is simply the awakening of one heart by another, of sincerity by sincerity. Although words can express it, and can point to it, they cannot substitute for it. It is the authentic experience which occurs when concern with all that is inessential drops away.
>
> (Brazier, 1995, pp. 12–13)

We would say that this is also a description of client-centred therapy in action; it too might be said to be the awakening of one heart by another, of the experience of being empathetically understood, unconditionally accepted, and genuinely received. Although often thought of as a Western therapy, we believe that client-centred therapy in practice has much in common with Eastern therapies, since it is based on reaching toward an authentic human relationship, and the notion that there is a tendency towards actualisation. As Hansard (2001) writes in his popular book, *The Tibetan Art of Living*:

> The seeds within the fruit only know one thing: that they must grow, blossom and bear fruit. Essentially, we human beings must do the same, but some of us have forgotten. The truth is everywhere, in all things, in all situations and is behind the beginning and completion of everything. It can lead you to your spiritual potential and, most of all, it can reveal to you how to live your own life.
>
> (Hansard, 2001, p. 19)

Existential psychotherapy

We have also seen how our perspective on positive therapy can allow for a range of techniques, but what is most important are the fundamental assumptions of the therapist and how they employ the techniques in the service of the client's organismic valuing process. In describing how other approaches might be considered under the umbrella of positive therapy, we are careful not to lose sight of this principle. At base, the approach we are describing is idiosyncratic to the relationship between the client and the therapist, and the task of the therapist is to help the client hear their own inner voice. Positive therapy is ultimately an existential endeavour:

> Radical existential psychotherapy focuses on the inter-personal and supra-personal dimensions, as it tries to capture and question people's worldviews. Such existential work aims at clarifying and understanding personal values and beliefs, making explicit what was previously implicit and unsaid. Its practice is primarily philosophical and seeks to enable a person to live more deliberately, more authentically and more purposefully, whilst accepting the limitations and contradictions of human existence . . . Existential psychotherapy has to be reinvented and recreated by every therapist and with every new client. It is essentially about investigating human existence and the particular preoccupations of one individual and this has to be done without preconceptions or set ways of proceeding. There has to be complete openness to the individual situation and an attitude of wonder that will allow the specific circumstances and experiences to unfold in their own right.
>
> (Deurzen, 1998, pp. 13–14)

Similarly, from an existential therapy background, Bretherton and Ørner (2003) write:

> [T]he most obvious way in which the existential approach parallels positive psychotherapy is in its preoccupation with what is presented by the client rather than with global models of deficit and disorder. Using the phenomenological method, therapists attempt to 'bracket' [put to one side] many of the assumptions and reactions they have with regard to clients (including the desire for therapeutic progress) so as to better engage with a client's way of being. By stepping back from their own prejudices and stereotypes, existential therapists can identify client's possibilities as well as their limitations . . . The existentialists suggest that by identifying the constellations of meaning by which we relate to the world, we give ourselves the opportunity of decision – to decide whether to alter our way of being in the world.
>
> (Bretherton & Ørner, 2003, p. 136)
> (see also Bretherton & Ørner, 2004)

Conclusion

In conclusion for this chapter, our stance is that it is not what the therapist *does* (i.e., their technique) that determines whether a therapy is a good candidate as a positive therapy. Rather it is what the therapist *thinks* (i.e., their fundamental assumptions), that is important. The crux of being a positive therapist is that the therapist adopts a way of thinking that fully embraces the notion that their task is to facilitate the client's actualising tendency. It is our ideas about human nature that make us the psychotherapists we are. As Yalom (2001) writes:

> When I was finding my way as a young psychotherapy student, the most useful book I read was Karen Horney's *Neurosis and Human Growth*. And the single most useful concept in that book was the notion that the human being has an inbuilt propensity toward self-realization. If obstacles are removed, Horney believed, the individual will develop into a mature, fully realized adult, just as an acorn will develop into an oak tree. 'Just as an acorn develops into an oak . . .' What a wonderful liberating and clarifying image! It forever changed my approach to psychotherapy by offering me a new vision of my work: My task was to remove obstacles blocking my patient's path. I did not have to do the entire job; I did not have to inspirit the patient with the desire to grow, with curiosity, will, zest for life, caring, loyalty, or any of the myriad of characteristics that make us fully human. No, what I had to do was to identify and remove obstacles. The rest would follow automatically, fueled by the self-actualizing forces within the patient.
>
> (Yalom, 2001, p. 1)

This quote from Yalom captures for us the essence of what we would call positive therapy. It is the client and not the therapist who knows best. But we would not want the reader to come away thinking that we are saying that the client's inner voice is easily articulated. On the contrary, it is a difficult path. Although there are a variety of new, pre-fabricated therapeutic approaches that embrace the ideas we have been discussing, what we find parti-cularly appealing are the person-centred therapies, as they are founded on the therapists principled use of the concept of the actualising tendency. Our understanding of Rogers' (1957, 1959) approach permits for a broad and flexible way of working that is individual to the client. It is about working in a way that is not wedded to the use of any one particular set of techniques, but rather the necessary and sufficient conditions provide an attitudinal base that underlies the therapist's approach to the relationship. Like Yalom (2001), we would advise against sectarianism and advocate therapeutic pluralism, but we would also stress that this therapeutic pluralism needs to be consistent with the therapist's underlying assumptions. Specifically within the sense of positive therapy, this means that the therapist can work as they consider to be appropriate, provided that they are always allowing articulation of the client's actualising tendency rather than imposing their own desires and agendas.

Chapter 5

Therapeutic process and positive psychological techniques

As positive psychologists, we are informed by person-centred theory. At the same time, as practitioners with an interest in the person-centred approach, we are informed by psychology, and strive to take a wider perspective on therapy. In the previous chapter, we discussed the family of person-centred therapies, and other approaches that in our view might be said to constitute positive therapies – insofar as the fundamental assumptions underlying practice remain the same, i.e., that the client is their own best expert. This is the crux of the idea of positive therapy as we see it.

Drawing on positive psychology research, there are a tremendous amount of intervention strategies that clients might sometimes find useful (see e.g., Linley & Joseph, 2004a; Lopez & Snyder, 2003). The use of intervention techniques is a contentious issue within client-centred therapy. However, we see no reason why positive therapists should not draw on the wider resources available to them, as long as they are able to articulate how the use of particular tests or techniques are helping to facilitate the client's OVP (see Bozarth, 1991). As Yalom (2001) writes:

> [T]he flow of therapy should be spontaneous, forever following unanticipated riverbeds: it is grotesquely distorted by being packaged into a formula . . . I try to avoid technique that is prefabricated and do best if I allow my choices to flow spontaneously.
>
> (Yalom, 2001, pp. 34–35)

Use of tests and measures

Positive psychology research tells us the importance of helping our clients realise their strengths. One of the debates in therapy is about how we actually go about doing this – how *do* we help people realise their strengths? This is where we as authors begin to differ. Although we both would describe ourselves as person centred in our philosophy, Stephen would describe himself as leaning toward what might be described as classical client-centred therapy, whereas Alex tends toward a more process-oriented approach. In large part, this may reflect our personalities and our understanding of person-centred psychology, but it also reflects the differences in the work we do.

Stephen would say that it is inevitable that in a therapeutic relationship in which the client feels valued, accepted, and not judged, that they will almost inevitably be drawn to exploring and understanding their strengths. As Peterson and Seligman (2003) describe, one's signature strengths convey a sense of ownership and authenticity, an intrinsic yearning to use them, and a feeling of inevitability in doing so. Using one's signature strengths is simply concordant with one's intrinsic interests and values, and hence within a supportive environmental context, the client's strengths will be recognised and become a topic of exploration. In many senses, one can understand Peterson and Seligman's description of strengths here as being an expression of what we would call, within person-centred theory, the actualising tendency.

Now this is not to say that when clients express an interest in learning about themselves in such a way that might be facilitated by the use of self-report questionnaires that Stephen would not use them. He would readily, so long as the agenda is about staying with the client and going in their direction. If the client expressed interest in learning more about themselves or about some aspect of their life it may be in keeping with the person-centred approach, for example, to tell the client about available self-report questionnaires with which to assess their character strengths, or to give information on a topic. What is important is that the use of tests or other techniques are used as an expression of the necessary and sufficient conditions (Rogers, 1957) that constitute the therapeutic relationship.

Alex tends to agree very much with the view that therapy will often provide the opportunity for people to learn about themselves, and their strengths. However, in the work that he does as an executive coach, clients are likely to have more straightforward goals that lend themselves more readily to the use of tests that can facilitate the goal striving process. It is also more likely to be the case that in executive coaching settings, the agenda is not so much about the client's self-discovery, but about their pursuit of organisational objectives. As such, the overall agenda here is not that of the client, but rather the organisation (and to confuse matters even further, it is often the organisation that is the paying client, rather than the individual being coached).

In a more process-oriented coaching setting the client (i.e., the coachee) may have as their agenda to be more successful in achieving their goals. If this is the case, Alex would be quite open to the use of personality and strengths assessments that could facilitate this process. However, the use of assessment in this way is underpinned by two important caveats. First, it is always the case that assessment is offered to the client as a suggestion that can be taken up or not, rather than prescribed by the 'coach as expert'. This is crucial, since it underpins the fundamental principle of the person-centred approach that we should be working to the client's agenda. Second, personality and strengths assessments are used in a facilitative way; they are not diagnostic. They open up areas for conversation and discussion, and can be swift and effective routes into those discussions. They are not used as ways of 'diagnosing', 'categorising', 'labelling', or otherwise imposing a 'coach as expert's' view on the person.

It is likely that there are differences here in the clients' agendas, with therapy clients being more interested in exploring themselves, their past, and their relation to the world with the aim of personal transformation, and coaching clients being more interested in understanding themselves but only to the extent that it gives them leverage in achieving their specific future-oriented goals. Further, it may be that it is these differences that would influence whether or not we might consider it appropriate to use a specific assessment in order to understand more about the client's strengths. Either way, both of us are in agreement that what is most important here is our respect for the client's agenda. Our professional practice would simply be ineffective, we believe, if we imposed our beliefs and values on our clients, rather than being guided by them and their actualising tendency. It is this shared deep philosophical assumption that unites us, but when it comes to specific therapies such as those discussed in the following section we would debate between us the extent to which our intention to follow the client's agenda is compromised by taking a process direction approach. But we do not want to raise this debate here, as this would detract us from our main purpose, which is to argue that positive psychological approaches to therapy adopt the person-centred meta-theoretical foundation to ground theory and practice.

Assessment and diagnosis

Many in the person-centred community object to the use of tests and measures, seeing their use as conflated with assessment and diagnosis (see Wilkins, 2005b). To the extent that such tests and measures are used to 'diagnose' and 'categorise' people, labelling them as suffering from this or that disorder, we agree. However, positive psychology research offers us a different repertoire of assessments, founded from different perspectives and outlooks, that do not require that people are 'diagnosed', 'categorised', or 'labelled'. Rather, as we have begun to illustrate, there are many tests and measures in positive psychology that clients may themselves find useful, such as assessing their strengths, and which may form the focus for collaboration in the therapy or coaching session.

Thus, we do not object to tests and measures per se. They have a number of uses. But we do both object to the idea of diagnosis and assessment from the perspective of the medical model. Given that person-centred theory holds that psychopathology develops as a result of internalised conditions of worth and that amelioration of psychopathology takes place when the right social environmental conditions are present, the approach to therapy remains the same regardless of what problem the person presents with. Thus, there is no need for diagnosis, in the medical model sense. Diagnosis is only necessary within the medical model, which holds that psychological problems like medical problems require specific diagnosis in order to determine the appropriate specific treatment.

Client-centred therapists therefore do not routinely take case histories, assess, or diagnose their clients, as they do not make the assumption that there are specific treatments for specific problems. As we saw in Chapter 4, psychological problems are as a result of the internalisation of conditions of worth. The client-centred therapist, in offering the core conditions to their client, is able to offer a social environment that serves to dissolve the client's conditions of worth. As the client begins to feel unconditionally accepted in the therapeutic relationship, perhaps for the first time in his or her life, he or she is able to begin to develop unconditional self-acceptance. With unconditional self-acceptance, the client is able to accurately

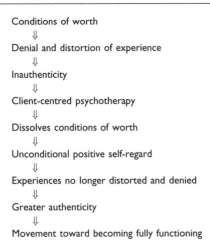

Conditions of worth
⇓
Denial and distortion of experience
⇓
Inauthenticity
⇓
Client-centred psychotherapy
⇓
Dissolves conditions of worth
⇓
Unconditional positive self-regard
⇓
Experiences no longer distorted and denied
⇓
Greater authenticity
⇓
Movement toward becoming fully functioning

Figure 5.1 Theoretical process of client-centred therapy

symbolise experience in awareness, and move toward an integration of self with experience. As the conditions of worth dissolve
incongruence between self and experience decreases and this results
in movement toward becoming more authentic and fully functioning (see Merry, 1999) (see Figure 5.1):

> The individual's return to unconditional positive self-regard is
> the crux of psychological growth in the theory. It is the factor
> that reunifies the self with the actualizing tendency . . . Rogers'
> hypothesises that one must perceive reception of uncondi-
> tional positive regard in order to correct the pathological state.
> The communication of unconditional positive regard by a
> significant other is one way to achieve the above conditions.
> (Bozarth, 1998, p. 84)

Client-centred therapists will differ in the extent to which they
hold that diagnosis, formulation, and assessment are unnecessary.
Most would, of course, agree with this position, that client-centred
therapy is a single approach to therapy regardless of the presenting
problem, but some will take different views on the use of diagnosis
and assessment, depending on their work context, or other cir-
cumstances (see Wilkins, 2005b). For instance, although we take
the view that person-centred theory is probably a much more

comprehensive theory in accounting for the range of psychopathology than is often thought, there are probably certain problems in living that do not result from the internalisation of conditions of worth. Maybe those problems often classified as psychosis or mania, for example, fall outside the spotlight of person-centred theory. We do not know for sure where the boundary lies, and for this reason we would caution against the disregard of the body of knowledge built up by psychologists and psychiatrists about the various so-called psychiatric disorders. But we also caution against the uncritical acceptance of the medical model.

We hope to have illustrated in our discussion of the use of tests and measures how we think that although person-centred practitioners are often set against the use of tests and measures – conflating their use with the medical model – there is no reason not to use tests and measures within the person-centred framework. The same goes for the variety of other therapeutic approaches that might also be said to constitute the positive therapies. What is important we think is the therapist's underlying philosophical stance – their fundamental assumptions – and therefore it is not what the therapist does that is important, it is *how* they do it. Many person-centred therapists are set against using techniques drawn from other therapy schools, such as the two-chair technique used by Gestalt therapists, or the use of cognitive-behavioural techniques, but what we would say is that there is nothing wrong with the use of any of these particular techniques per se. What is wrong is that often they are employed by people whose fundamental assumptions are that they, and not the client themselves, are the client's best expert. We do object to this assumption, but we see no reason to object to the use of such techniques by therapists who deeply hold the core philosophical stance that the client is their own best expert. Thus, there are a range of other therapies and techniques that the more process-oriented and integrative therapist might draw on (see Worsley, 2001, 2004), and we go on to illustrate some of these now.

Process orientation

The following is not meant in any way as a comprehensive list, but as a brief excursion into some of the other therapies and techniques that we find interesting and useful ourselves. At this point we think it is useful again to emphasise what we consider would constitute a 'positive therapy' from our understanding. The defining feature of 'positive therapy', we would argue, is that the therapist holds with the idea that the client is their own best expert and possesses within them an innate developmental tendency toward growth and fulfilment. As such, this means in practice that the therapist should always be following the client's agenda, and seeking to promote their actualising tendency, rather than considering themselves as the 'expert' on the client, and thereby imposing their 'expertise' on the client.

Considered in this way, 'positive therapy' permits a very broad range of therapeutic techniques. It also offers a meta-theory that carries across a whole variety of contexts in which one person may work to facilitate the growth and development of another. We have noted already how Alex's executive coaching work is premised on his theoretical assumptions about the actualising tendency, and we have considered very briefly how these ideas might be used in practice in his coaching work. We now consider some other approaches that offer techniques to the more process-oriented coach or therapist.

Transactional analysis

Eric Berne (1910–1970) introduced a system of therapy known as transactional analysis (TA). Stewart (1989), a leading exponent of TA and of Berne's work, says that the practice of TA is founded on three assumptions. The first of these is that at their core people are 'OK'. Although the therapist may not like the person's behaviour, the therapist values and esteems the client. Second, the TA therapist holds that each person has the capacity to think and make decisions about their life. Third, people can behave differently: how we think, feel, and behave is our own choice. These assumptions are consistent with the values of person-centred theory that we described earlier, and some person-centred practitioners adopt an integrative approach to their work that draws heavily on the ideas of TA (e.g., Worsley, 2001). As such, we will explore the principles and uses of TA in some more depth.

Thinking Martian

One of things Berne encouraged people to do was to think 'Martian': to be able to observe human behaviour without preconceptions about what it means, to listen to *how* people say things as well as *what* they say. This involves the recognition that messages from one person to another can operate on two levels, which Berne referred to as the social level and the psychological level. The social level refers to what we say to one another whereas the psychological level refers to what we really mean. For example, at a social level we might greet someone with the words, 'It's nice to see you', but the tone of our voice, or our eye contact, might say something else, such as 'Oh no, I was hoping you wouldn't be here, it really isn't nice to see you at all'. When the social and the psychological levels are incongruent in this way, the psychological message is said to be *ulterior*. Berne maintained that the psychological message was always the real message, and it was at this psychological level that the course of events was always determined. People would act in ways that were guided by their real values, motives, and intentions, not by those values, motives, and intentions that they pretended to hold. In practice, the role of the TA therapist is to be aware of, and to help the client become aware of, the psychological level in his or her communication. One way to do this is through teaching the client about ego states.

Ego states

Berne outlined a complex theoretical framework that therapists use to discuss the nature of interpersonal communication with clients. He outlined what he called the ego state model. This consists of three ego states: the child, the parent, and the adult. In our child ego state, we think and feel in a way like we did when we were children. In our parent ego state, we think and feel in a way like those of the significant parental figures from our childhood. In our adult ego state, we think and feel in ways that are direct responses to the here and now environment. Parental states can be nurturing or controlling, and child states can be free or adapted. The nurturing parent corresponds to those aspects of parenting activity that have promoted growth and fostered autonomy. The controlling parent is the voice that criticises behaviour. The free child is closely related to contact with the organismic valuing process. The adapted child stems from times when we had to adapt our behaviour in response to the demands of others (i.e., their conditions of worth). Any behaviour is driven by the ego state that is in control of the personality at that moment.

Feelings of inferiority as well as those of spontaneous joy are associated with the child. Criticism and orthodoxy are associated with the parent. Unemotional appraisal of the environment is associated with the adult. Normally we move in and out of these different ego states and psychopathology could be understood in terms of the functional breakdown of barriers between ego states. For example, delusional ideation occurs where there is a breakdown between child and adult ego states such that child imagery contaminates the adult appraisal of the world. We can also analyse interpersonal interactions in terms of the communication between individuals at an ego state level of analysis. Often, at a social level, it might appear that we are talking adult to adult, but at the psychological level, something else is happening. For example, we are talking parent to child, or child to parent. Berne also described the pathological games that people play in terms of stereotyped ego state communication. By introducing our clients to the language of ego states, they can become empowered to explore their own issues from this new perspective. Consider the following example:

Teresa goes to see a therapist because she often has problems with her line manager at work. Her line manager is a middle-aged man and Teresa is a young woman in her twenties. Teresa experiences her line manager as very controlling. In meetings, she often finds herself becoming confused and feeling patronised. She feels angry but tries to hide her anger, becoming tearful, often causing problems among her team workers who can't understand Teresa's reactions. During one session, Teresa mentioned that when she was a student she had read the book by Eric Berne, *Games People Play*, which one of her flatmates had had. This opened up conversation in this direction and the therapist offered to say a bit more about the ideas of Eric Berne, which Teresa welcomed. Through the TA framework, Teresa began to understand how her line manager spoke to her at the social level as adult to adult, but further exploration showed how at the ulterior level he would be communicating from parent to her child, leaving Teresa confused and bewildered. As Teresa began to realise this, she felt empowered in her interactions and began to explore new ways of remaining in the adult ego state when her line manager invited her into the child ego state.

Life script

Transactional analysis provides a very elaborate model of psycho-pathology, taking the view that psychological problems often have their roots in childhood. Understanding our communication with others also involves exploring the client's life script. This is the plan decided in early life by each person about the course of their life, how it begins, what happens in the middle, and how it ends. The life script is likened to each person's own unfolding drama. Berne said that the life script was laid down between the ages of 3 and 7, and reflects one of four possible judgements about the self and others:

1   I'm OK and you're OK.
2   I'm not OK, but you're OK.
3   I'm OK, but you're not OK.
4   I'm not OK, and you're not OK.

Such feelings reflect parental introjections in infancy, and form the basis of how the child experiences his or her life. As the introjection of these parental messages takes place at such a young age, they are not the product of reasoned and logical thinking. In childhood, each of us develops our own personal life story, which is referred to as the life script. We carry these life scripts into adulthood and play them out unconsciously, finding ways to confirm our early decisions. The content of our scripts is unique to each of us, although common script themes have been identified. For example:

I mustn't grow up.
I mustn't be important.
I mustn't exist.
I mustn't make it.
I mustn't be important.
I mustn't feel.
I mustn't be me.

The therapist endeavours to identify the client's beliefs about their life script and to confront the life script and encourage autonomy. The therapist aims to facilitate the client's recognition that they can now make different decisions in life (see Stewart,

1989). The life script represents the infant's way of surviving and getting their needs met in what seems to be a hostile world. The child makes decisions, at an unconscious level, and as an adult the person plays out part of this script. For example, the child might perceive the parent as wanting them to be different. With parents who wanted a girl instead of a boy, for example, a child might come to decide that 'I mustn't be me'. This script belief might be expressed in a variety of ways, for example, a sense of the self as inferior, or through behaviour typical of the opposite sex. This is, of course, similar to the idea of conditions of worth from the person-centred approach, although clients may find the ideas of a life script easier to understand and relate to. Transactional analysis offers techniques and ways of thinking that can be useful to clients in thinking about how problems in living arose and are maintained in everyday life, but it offers a way of working with people that is not just about alleviating psychopathology, but about becoming more self-determining in life and able to make new decisions toward more optimal functioning.

Although transactional analysis has a wide appeal, and is popular as a therapy approach and in group and management training, it has not been subject to extensive scientific testing as a form of therapy. Although as positive therapists we might find TA appealing because of the shared fundamental assumptions, and we might find some of the metaphorical ideas of TA useful in talking with our clients, we must remember that it remains an underresearched approach. Nonetheless, for experiential work it provides a rich source of material for those therapists whose approach to their work is more process driven (e.g., Worsley, 2001, 2004).

Early views of positive therapy and positive clinical psychology

In addition to these well-established therapeutic techniques drawn from TA, there are a number of other therapeutic approaches that we think share many of the same positive psychology assumptions. It is important to note that although we have talked here about client-centred therapy as a form of positive therapy, we would not want to prescribe what it is to be a positive therapist in terms of what the therapist says or does. Other therapeutic approaches that also emphasise the client as the active agent might be equally good candidates as positive therapies (see, for example, Follette,

Linnerooth, & Ruckstuhl, 2001; Resnick, Warmoth, & Serlin, 2001). In the sections that follow, we will briefly describe some of the therapeutic approaches that might be considered from a positive therapy perspective. This may be because they have evolved explicitly from a positive psychology tradition, or because they draw on positive psychological constructs, processes, or techniques. Again, we emphasise that what constitutes positive therapy, for us, is the therapist's fundamental assumption and deep-seated belief in the actualising tendency of the client. Provided that the therapist holds with this assumption, and works to facilitate the client's natural developmental propensities, then positive therapy permits of a wide variety of therapeutic techniques.

Seligman (2002) and Seligman and Peterson (2003) have discussed what they see as positive therapy and positive clinical psychology. Their central contention is that much of what makes therapy successful is what they refer to as the 'deep strategies', such as instilling hope, providing narration, and building strengths, all of which are employed, instinctively and intuitively, by successful therapists. However, the problem arises, they suggest, in that these deep strategies are not named or specifically recognised, and hence they are not researched, trained for, or developed (see also Maddux et al., 2004b, and our discussion of 'positive clinical psychology' in Chapter 6). We would agree with this statement when it comes to mainstream professional psychology trainings in clinical and counselling psychology. However, this is only true to a lesser extent in those trainings with a person-centred leaning, because it is implicit in the person-centred approach that the deep strategies are already within the client themselves. As such, the therapist is trained to help facilitate the client in developing their own instinct and intuition, so that they are able to heal themselves and find their own best directions in life.

Motivational interviewing

Another more recent approach often used in health psychology contexts is that of motivational interviewing (Rollnick & Miller, 1995). Motivational interviewing was based on the finding that the person-centred qualities of the therapist were important ingredients of therapy. However, motivational interviewing adds a more process-directive element by skilfully helping the client to explore the pros and cons of change in order to motivate the client towards making the necessary changes. Motivational interviewing has been described as a brief and directive technique driven form of person-centred therapy.

Solution-focused therapy

Solution-focused therapy is claimed to be unique, because its focus is on the client's solutions, rather than their problems (O'Connell, 2005). It is based on helping clients to achieve their preferred outcomes through the evocation and co-construction of solutions to their problems (O'Connell, 2001). Solution-focused therapy arose from the work of Steve de Shazer and his team at the Brief Family Therapy Center in Milwaukee, in the United States, on brief therapy. While there is some debate as to what constitutes 'brief therapy', there is an emerging consensus that brief therapy involves fewer than 20 sessions (O'Connell, 2005).

There is considerable agreement about what the main characteristics of brief therapy are, and perusing them shows their commonality with much of what we are describing within the framework of positive therapy. For example, Barret-Kruse (1994) summarised some of the main features of solution-focused brief therapy as the view that oneself and others are essentially able; the therapist's acceptance of the client's definition of the problem; the formation of the therapeutic alliance; and the client being credited for therapeutic success, while the therapist also learns from the client. She does also suggest that this process requires a degree of directivity from the therapist, thus locating this approach among the more process-oriented positive therapies that we are describing.

Positive psychotherapy (PPT)

PPT is a manualised six-week intervention consisting of six one and a half hour sessions based on Seligman's (2003b) theory of authentic happiness (Parks, 2004). It is prescriptive, and involves the client engaging in various exercises over the six weeks. For example, in week 1 the client is asked to tell a story about them at their best, and to complete a questionnaire to assess their strengths, and to think of ways in which to use their strengths more often (Parks, 2004). The theoretical rationale underpinning this is that using one's strengths conveys a sense of ownership and authenticity in their use, because people feel an intrinsic yearning to use them and a feeling of inevitability in doing so. Hence, using one's signature strengths is considered to be concordant with one's intrinsic interests and values (Peterson & Seligman, 2004). Although not explicitly stated, one can see how signature strengths could be seen as representative of the actualising tendency: they are entirely consistent with who we are as individuals, we feel drawn to using our strengths, doing so intrinsically and for the fulfilment that they provide. Further, Peterson and Seligman suggest that the use of strengths will bring about tangible outcomes, such as subjective well-being, competence, efficacy, mastery, mental health, and rich social networks. Hence, using one's signature strengths is considered to serve well-being and basic psychological needs, such as competence, autonomy, relatedness, and self-esteem. In this way, using one's strengths is considered to act as a buffer against mental illness (Seligman & Peterson, 2003). Although in its early stages, preliminary evidence from the PPT research programme suggests that this is an effective way of helping people with mild depression (Parks, 2004). Further, more recent work is beginning to provide evidence for a range of exercises that can simultaneously increase happiness and decrease depression. These include using your signature strengths in a new way, and counting one's blessings by thinking about three good things, and their causes, that had happened each day (Seligman et al., 2005).

We should also note here that 'positive psychotherapy' has been developed by Peseschkian and colleagues (e.g., Peseschkian & Tritt, 1998). However, this approach is not drawn from the positive psychology tradition, but instead notes that the 'positive' in its title is drawn from the word '"positum", i.e., from what is factual and given' (Peseschkian & Tritt, 1998, p. 94). Hence, while its title may be misleading to a modern audience, given more recent developments within positive psychology and the advent of 'positive therapy' and 'positive psychotherapy' from the positive psychological tradition, we would not consider Peseschkian's 'positive psychotherapy' to be a positive psychotherapy within the positive psychological sense.

Well-being therapy

Well-being therapy was developed by Fava and colleagues (e.g., Fava, 1997, 1999; Ruini & Fava, 2004), based on Ryff's (e.g., 1989; Ryff & Singer, 1996) research on the six identified domains of psychological well-being, namely environmental mastery, personal growth, purpose in life, autonomy, self-acceptance, and positive relations with others. Well-being therapy is described as a short-term psychotherapeutic strategy that extends over eight sessions, with each session ranging from 30 to 50 minutes. It emphasises self-observation, including the use of a structured diary, and the interaction between the client and the therapist (Ruini & Fava, 2004, p. 374).

Fava (2000) recognised that cognitive-behavioural therapies had impressive track records in symptom reduction, but were lacking in their complete resolution of psychopathology. Ruini and Fava (2004) identified four reasons that provided the context for the development of well-being therapy. First, there has been increasing awareness of relapse in affective disorders, especially unipolar major depression. While therapeutic intervention may remove the symptoms for a time, the effects are not particularly long lasting. Second, concerns of residual symptomatology, such as anxiety, irritability, and interpersonal problems, have often been found to characterise patients who were in remission according to DSM criteria, but who were nonetheless still far from well-functioning. Third, increasing interest in quality of life assessment in healthcare has placed these questions more squarely on the clinical agenda. Fourth, the growth of positive psychology has brought to bear positive psychological perspectives on clinical populations, further driving the need for the promotion of well-being, rather than just the alleviation of symptomatology.

Recognising this, Fava (e.g., 1999) sought to build on existing cognitive-behavioural frameworks but also to incorporate a focus on the facilitation of well-being, in the belief that improvements in well-being would serve to buffer against subsequent psycho-pathology, thereby countering relapse, reducing residual symptom-atology, and improving global functioning and psychological well-being. Using Ryff's framework of psychological well-being (e.g., Ryff & Singer, 1996), which includes the six dimensions of environmental mastery, personal growth, purpose in life, auton-omy, self-acceptance, and positive relations with others, the client is helped to identify areas of their psychological well-being that may be improved. The therapist then proceeds to work with the client on these areas, as well as on the presenting symptoms of disorder.

During the initial session, the client is asked to identify episodes of well-being and locate them in their situational context, no matter how short lived they were. During the intermediate sessions, the client is encouraged to identify the thoughts and beliefs that lead to the premature interruption of well-being, but with the trigger for self-observation being based on well-being, rather than distress. The therapist uses this information to identify specific impairments in well-being, and then works with the client to repair these. The therapist may also choose to use self-rating inventories, such as Ryff's (1989) psychological well-being scales, to assist with the identification of problematic well-being areas. This information then paves the way for more specific well-being enhancement strategies (for a fuller discussion, see Ruini & Fava, 2004).

To date, well-being therapy has been used very effectively with people suffering from a range of clinical disorders, including affective disorders (Fava, Rafanelli, Cazzaro, Conti, & Grandi, 1998a), recurrent depression (Fava, Rafanelli, Grandi, Conti, & Belluardo, 1998b), loss of clinical effect (Fava, Ruini, Rafanelli, & Grandi, 2002), and generalized anxiety disorder (Fava et al., 2005).

Mindfulness-based cognitive therapy

Mindfulness has long been recognised as a means for improving self-awareness, and thereby allowing one to make more informed and deliberate choices. Recent empirical work from the positive psychology tradition has shown how mindfulness is associated with a host of well-being indicators (Brown & Ryan, 2003). It has also been shown that mindfulness-based approaches provide possible means of fostering self-determination and self-awareness, and in this way allow the satisfaction of basic psychological needs for autonomy, competence and relatedness (see Brown & Ryan, 2003, 2004), which are believed to underpin much of human well-being (Ryan & Deci, 2000).

Within therapeutic settings, mindfulness training has been allied with cognitive-behavioural therapy in order to try and prevent the problems of relapse following treatment for depression that were described earlier. According to Teasdale, Segal, Williams, Ridgeway, Soulsby, & Law (2000), vulnerability to relapse and recurrence of depression arises from the fact that the person makes repeated associations between their depressed mood and patterns of negative, self-devaluing, hopeless thinking during episodes of major depression. This leads to changes at both the cognitive and neuronal levels, such that people who have experienced major depression, but who have recovered, differ from people who have never experienced major depression in their patterns of thinking that are triggered by low mood or dysphoria.

The focus of mindfulness-based cognitive therapy is then to teach individuals to become aware of how thoughts and feelings relate to them in a wider, decentred perspective. In this way, people are encouraged to view their thoughts as 'mental events' that are detached from, rather than an integral part of, the person and their psychological make-up. This detachment then provides individuals with the skills and abilities they need in order to prevent the escalation of depressive thoughts and feelings into full-blown major depression. There is growing evidence to support the effectiveness of this approach (see e.g., Ma & Teasdale, 2004; Teasdale, Moore, Hayhurst, Pope, Williams, & Segal, 2002) and for its use with a variety of clinical as well as non-clinical conditions (Grossman, Niemann, Schmidt, & Walach, 2004).

Clinical approaches to posttraumatic growth

In our own work, we have been concerned with the concept of posttraumatic growth, or how people change and grow positively following trauma. In thinking about how clinicians may work with people following trauma in such a way that promotes and facilitates the person's capacity for growth and positive change, Tedeschi and Calhoun (2004; Calhoun & Tedeschi, 1999) are explicit in noting that therapy that seeks to facilitate posttraumatic growth is always client led, moving at the client's pace and in the client's direction. The therapist acts as a co-traveller who, when appropriate, may note certain developments or offer alternative interpretations.

Tedeschi and Calhoun (2004) suggest six general considerations for the therapist to bear in mind when working to facilitate posttraumatic growth. These are very much consistent with our understanding of positive therapy, and so we will elaborate them a little here. First, Tedeschi and Calhoun remind the therapist that they should be working from the framework of the trauma survivor, striving to understand the client's way of thinking rather than imposing their own views, values, and beliefs. Second, they commend the value of effective listening, and suggest that the therapist should listen without necessarily trying to resolve the client's issues for them. Third, they suggest the therapist listens for and labels the themes of posttraumatic growth, but always with this process being led by the client, rather than directed by the therapist. Fourth, the therapist should focus on the struggle rather than the trauma; the growth that may come is a result of this struggle and adaptation, rather than a result of the trauma per se. Fifth, trauma survivors may be able to learn much from others who have experienced similar events, and, as such, group approaches to the facilitation of posttraumatic growth merit consideration (see the consideration of these in Chapter 7). Finally, helping the client to engage with a developing narrative about their struggle, and to monitor their changing beliefs following the trauma can act as triggers for the recognition and celebration of growth, but as ever, only if done at the client's pace and from the client's perspective (see Tedeschi & Calhoun, 2004, for further elaboration).

While there are not yet empirical data to support clinical approaches to the facilitation of posttraumatic growth, these therapeutic positions are very much concordant with how we would understand positive therapy. Indeed, elsewhere in our work (Joseph, 2004; Joseph & Linley, 2005b), we have elaborated on a person-centred organismic valuing theory of how people adapt positively following stressful and traumatic events, and this provides a solid foundation from which to develop a more specified positive psychological therapy for the facilitation of growth following trauma. This is something to which we return in Chapter 7.

Domains of resource

In adopting an integrated approach there is a vast wealth of theory and technique available. We can think of interventions as reflecting the various domains of resource that a person can tap into, i.e., physical, environmental, relational, feelings, effective thinking, continuity of past and present, and transcendence through spirituality. Kauffman (2005) has clients use the mnemonic of 'perfect' to remind themselves to scan through these seven resources in order to stimulate possible ideas of what might help when they need more psychological energy to move forward. She gives the example of how she uses these resources when clients are feeling thwarted on their quest toward their goals.

When working with a student or author experiencing writer's block, for example, she would help them assess if there is a physical component to the challenge, or a physical intervention that will foster their capacity to write (e.g., improve nutrition, take a nap, go for a swim). Are there resources in the environment the client could access or ways the immediate environment could be changed (e.g., visit a website community for advice, or go the library today instead)? What about relations (e.g., talk to someone)? What about feelings (e.g., take time out to read some jokes to increase positive mood or mindfully metabolise anxiety). What about effective thinking (e.g., is the block a result of getting stuck into too much detail)? What about the continuity of past/present/future (e.g., tapping into life lessons learned in the past, mindfulness or optimism exercises)? What about transcendence through spirituality (e.g., put on contemplative music)?

What Kauffman (2005) emphasises is the importance of holistic approach to our work. Working in an integrative manner allows for broader focus and prevents us and our clients to become entrenched in one single approach. Reminding them of the multiple resources and approaches possible increases a sense of agency and multiple pathways, the core skills that foster hope (Snyder, 2000).

Conclusion

In this chapter, we have discussed how the use of tests and measures is controversial in the context of person-centred therapy when they are used from the perspective of the medical model. In person-centred therapy, there is no need to diagnosis or assess from the perspective of the medical model as it is thought that no matter what the presenting condition, it is the therapeutic relationship that is healing in all cases. However, as positive therapists we argue that tests and measures, particularly those derived from the positive psychology perspective, can often be useful in the context of therapy in helping the client's own self-understanding. But what is important is that the use of tests and measures are used from the client's frame of reference so that they remain their own best expert. Similarly, although the use of various psychological techniques is controversial among many client-centred therapists, there are a variety of existing techniques and therapeutic approaches, such as transactional analysis, motivational interviewing, and solution-focused therapy, which the more process-directed therapist may find helpful. Positive psychologists too have begun to explore and develop new ways of working, and we described four rapidly developing areas of work: well-being therapy developed by Fava and his colleagues, positive psychotherapy and happiness interventions, mindfulness-based cognitive therapy, and clinical approaches to posttraumatic growth. It is our expectation that coming years will see a mushrooming of further interest in these therapies. We discuss these therapeutic techniques by way of example of the various forms of therapy that might be employed. But we emphasise that this book is not about technique, it is about reevaluating our fundamental assumptions as therapists, so that we use tests and techniques from a well-articulated philosophical perspective. As Rollo May (1994), one of the founding fathers of existential therapy, writes:

> Our Western tendency has been to believe that *understanding follows technique*; if we get the right technique, then we can penetrate the riddle of the patient, or, as said popularly with amazing perspicacity, we can 'get the other person's number'. The existential approach holds the exact opposite; namely, that *technique follows understanding*. The central task of the therapist is to seek to understand the patient as a being and as being-in-his-world. All technical problems are subordinate to this understanding. Without this understanding, technical facility is at best irrelevant, at worst a method of 'structuralizing' the neurosis. With it, the groundwork is laid for the therapist's being able to help the patient recognize and experience his own existence, and this is the central process of therapy. This does not derogate disciplined technique; it rather puts it into perspective.
>
> (May, 1994, p. 77)

Our view in this book is that what is important is the metatheoretical person-centred assumption that the client is their own best expert, and the idea that within each person there is an intrinsic motivation towards growth and optimal functioning. A variety of ways of working can coexist around this theoretical assumption.

Chapter 6

From psychopathology to well-being

In Chapters 4 and 5, we described our positive therapy approach as being founded on the person-centred theory of Carl Rogers, but one that is open to consideration of more process-driven work, drawing on ideas and using techniques drawn from other compatible approaches. The central thesis of the person-centred approach is that people have deep-seated innate propensities towards the actualisation of their potentialities, which can be either facilitated or impeded by the social environment. We also explored other therapeutic approaches that we think share this underlying assumption about human nature, and that might also be viewed under the umbrella of the positive therapies.

However, our emphasis on helping people to achieve their full potential and optimal functioning might lead some to think that these positive therapies are only for those who are already relatively well-functioning, and that people with more deep-seated issues and psychological problems would be best advised to seek help from more traditional psychological therapists. The reader will be aware that we have not provided an extensive discussion in this book on the various so-called psychiatric disorders. This is not because what we have to say cannot speak to the depths of human suffering, but because the approach we adopt rests on the assumption of the actualising tendency, which is an alternative paradigm to that of the medical model. In this chapter, we will demonstrate that our positive therapy approach is also relevant for helping us to understand psychopathology. We will go on to argue that person-centred theory and positive therapy provide alternatives to the medical model of psychopathology in the ways in which we conceptualise and understand people's psychological problems. This is what makes person-centred theory, and positive therapy, genuinely positive psychological theories of mental health (see also Joseph & Worsley, 2005a).

Integration of the positive and the negative

As we have seen in Chapter 1, positive psychology came about in response to the predominant late twentieth-century orientation of mainstream psychology to disease and the medical model. As such, it is entirely understandable that in this early phase of its history, there was the need for an emphasis on what was different about this approach, i.e., the focus on the positive. However, five years on, the pendulum has now swung away from an exclusive focus on the positive, and is resting at the place of a more integrative approach that includes both the positive and negative aspects of human functioning. This represents the idea of synthesis in Hegel's (1807/1931) work on the development of ideas as they move from *thesis* (i.e., traditional mainstream psychology) to *antithesis* (i.e., positive psychology), to *synthesis* (i.e., the integration with which we are now concerned).

As such, positive psychology's current position accords with calls for a new integrative psychology (Sternberg & Grigorenko, 2001). Thus, it is important that when we talk about positive therapy it is explicitly a therapy that speaks to both the negative and the positive aspects of human experience. At present there is no generally accepted meta-theory of positive psychology that helps to support this call for integration. However, we propose that person-centred personality theory provides an underlying meta-theory of personality development and mental health functioning, one that we have elaborated under the framework of positive therapy as being a meta-theoretical approach to positive psychological practice.

Person-centred psychopathology

We have already begun to explore psychopathology from the perspective of person-centred personality theory in previous chapters, and elsewhere (Joseph & Worsley, 2005a), showing how problems in living are thought to result from the internalisation of conditions of worth, which in turn thwart and usurp the actualising tendency, leading people to use this propensity towards development to self-actualise in a way consistent with their conditions of worth rather than congruently with their actualising tendency.

But can this theory really account for the range of problems people experience? Our view is that person-centred theory provides a much more comprehensive account of psychopathology than is generally recognised, and that it provides a powerful alternative to the medical model. This might surprise some people, as a common criticism of person-centred theory is that it is only concerned with the worried well, and that it fails to provide an explanation for severe and enduring psychological problems.

However, person-centred personality theory does account for our understanding of many severe and enduring psychological problems when the role of the distorted actualising tendency is fully and properly understood (see Wilkins, 2005a). For example, for some people, the theory suggests, the actualising tendency is thwarted and usurped to such a large extent that it would seem that there is nothing positive in the person, but that they are driven by a force for destruction. People still need to find outlets and expression for their directional tendencies (i.e., actualising tendency), but these directional tendencies have become warped and distorted through having to live within the confines and expectations of others (i.e., conditions of worth), rather than being able to develop in the directions that are congruent with their intrinsic values. As such, the person driven by extrinsic values reacts in negative and destructive ways, in an attempt to achieve conditional positive regard, rather than feeling free to pursue their own intrinsic directions, which, the theory argues, would be socially constructive and positive. The greater the mismatch (i.e. incongruence) between people's directions and the directions of their actualising tendency, the greater the extent of their psychopathology (see Wilkins, 2005a).

Thus, the fact that people behave in various ways that might be described as destructive is not evidence that falsifies person-centred theory, because the theory does not say, as some critics mistakenly believe, that people are always good. That would indeed be a most naïve position, as the critics say. However, what person-centred theory, as we have seen, says, is that people have an intrinsic motivation to develop in a constructive social direction, but that this motivation can be thwarted and usurped towards the fulfilment of conditions of worth. Hence, destructiveness arises when people actualise in the directions that are wrong for them, as the result of conditions of worth imposed from externally.

Thus, person-centred theory is able to provide an explanation for the suffering people have inflicted on one another. But we can also understand that it seems hard to grasp that, for example, some of the more destructive behaviours of humans simply came about through this process of internalisation of conditions of worth. Maybe, as some would suggest, the assumption that human nature consists of an intrinsic force towards actualisation is just wrong for some people. Maybe some people just do not have a tendency towards actualisation. We have heard colleagues in clinical psychology take this view, and say that some people are just born 'wired up' differently with no tendency toward actualisation, or in the popular press we read of people who are described as 'evil'. Their tendency is towards destruction. There are, of course, issues around the use of the word evil as a way of distancing ourselves from the humanity of the perpetrator (Worsley, 2005), but insofar as the use of such language is to describe extremes of behaviour, we are of the view that critics of person-centred personality theory have misunderstand the subtle and pervasive influence of conditions of worth, and how easily the actualising tendency can be thwarted, usurped, and thrown off course, with the result that it appears, developmentally, that the person is intrinsically motivated towards 'evil', and destructive behaviour. As Frankel and Sommerbeck (2005) write:

> Rogers' unconditional positive regard for a particular client emanates from his view that it is in the nature of human beings to be creative and constructive members of a society that offers each individual the greatest scope for self-expression. In this view, when an individual such as Hitler emerges, it is because his innate pro-social nature has been corrupted, just as a once friendly dog might become vicious on getting rabies. If young Adolf knew better he would not have *chosen* to be HITLER, the icon of evil, any more than a healthy dog would choose to become rabid.
>
> (Frankel & Sommerbeck, 2005, pp. 46–47)

Person-centred personality theory describes a very subtle developmental process. A very gentle touch of the rudder at an early stage will take the boat to a very different destination at the end of a long journey, and conditions of worth are similarly influential on the course of a person's life. Thus, in our view, it is not the case that the theory is lacking, or that we need to look elsewhere for an explanation of extreme human behaviour. Person-centred theory is robust enough to account for 'evil' behaviour, and that critics who see the presence of 'evil' behaviour as evidence against person-centred theory have simply misunderstood the subtle and profound nature of the theory.

Equally, it is not surprising that the person-centred theory is often misunderstood because it offers a radical alternative paradigm to much of the training in clinical and counselling psychology programmes, which adopt the medical model paradigm. Many in the field of clinical and counselling psychology are shocked when we say this, and respond that they do not adopt the medical model. They then go on to tell us how they do not view psychological problems as biological or genetic. But this is to misunderstand what is meant by the medical model.

By medical model, what we mean is the idea that the medical practitioner sets out to identify the problem and to prescribe a specific treatment. This is indeed what much of the training in clinical and counselling psychology does. A quick glance through many of the leading textbooks in the area show that chapters are set out to describe in turn each of the so-called psychiatric disorders, e.g., depression, anxiety, schizophrenia, obsessive compulsions, posttraumatic stress, and so on, with each of the chapters providing an account of the best preferred treatments for each. This is the medical model – the idea that there are specific problems requiring specific treatments. When we go to see the medical practitioner with a broken leg, we do not want her to give us tablets for indigestion, we want her to fix our broken leg. We want the appropriate treatment for our specific problem. The idea behind the textbooks in clinical psychology that lay out the chapters by so-called 'disorder' are no different from this – their task is also to ask what is the specific treatment needed for this specific disorder. In this chapter, we will argue that although sometimes the medical model may be appropriate for understanding human suffering, it has become too pervasive a way of understanding psychological suffering, and one which has misled many psychologists into believing that psychological problems are analogous to medical problems. But let us also be clear that in rejecting the medical model, we are explicitly not rejecting the idea of human suffering – only one particular view of how human suffering ought to be understood.

There is no doubt that psychological problems can become overwhelming in intensity and duration, causing a person to behave in extremely dysfunctional and dangerous ways, and in ways which are unusual for this person, or unusual for the society he or she lives in. As we have seen, we might define such experiences as psychopathology. We are not saying that psychopathology does not exist. Of course it does – the suffering of many people is all too real. The question is about how we understand psychopathology. We believe that we do ourselves a disservice as therapists in too readily adopting the medical model. What person-centred theory says is that these various forms of psychopathology, depression, anxiety, and so on, can be understood as ways in which people have developed as a result of their conditions of worth. Thus, all psychological problems are essentially the same: they are all individual expressions of incongruence between self and experience, and as a result there is no need for specific treatments (see Bozarth, 1998).

Redefining psychopathology: A positive psychology of mental health

Psychopathology therefore is a term that we will use to refer to thoughts, feelings, and behaviours that stem from our inner incongruence. This is a person-centred definition, and is different to the way in which many people think about psychopathology. As we have seen, mainstream approaches to psychology and psychiatry adopt the Diagnostic and Statistical Manual (DSM) of Mental Disorders (e.g., American Psychiatric Association, 2000), as a way of cataloguing the various ways in which psychopathology is expressed. These two systems are not incompatible, one can understand many of the various expressions of psychopathology listed in DSM as stemming from incongruence, but the person-centred approach also raises some other questions about psychopathology. The first of these is that the term psychopathology is used much more broadly to refer to behaviour and is not a term confined to use with people whose behaviours are extreme.

Continuity versus discontinuity

Certainly psychopathology is a term that refers to a range of seemingly very different psychological problems. One of the tasks of modern psychiatry and psychology has been to try and define various forms of psychopathology, and psychiatrists have produced a classification system containing hundreds of so-called psychiatric disorders (the Diagnostic and Statistical Manual of Mental Disorders; American Psychiatric Association, 2000).

However, although there are advantages to understanding psychopathology in this way, the classification of psychiatric disorders remains controversial and it is very difficult to draw a clear line between 'normality' and 'abnormality', to be able to say where psychopathology begins. How emotionally distressed or dysfunctional does a person have to be to be considered as suffering from a psychopathology? How long does emotional distress or dysfunction have to last, and how severe does it have to be, for it to be considered as psychopathology? In certain situations it would seem to be perfectly normal to be emotionally distressed, for example, when we are anxious in response to some threat or when we are sad in response to some loss. It is not unusual to be anxious before taking an important exam or to feel sadness at the loss of a loved one. But what of someone who always feels nervous when going into new social situations or someone who remains grieving for years after their loss? Would we say that these are examples of psychopathology?

Answers to such questions will often depend on which perspective is taken on the nature of psychological suffering. Certainly, problems in living are widespread. Nelson-Jones (1984), for example, draws attention to the difficulties experienced by the majority of people, how most of us struggle to be autonomous in how we live, and how Maslow (1970) used the term 'psychopathology of the average' to describe most people's level of functioning. We do not use the term psychopathology to refer only to the extremes of human behaviour, although of course at the extremes psychopathology is more evident. When we use the term 'psychopathology', we do so in recognising that within the person-centred model, all thoughts, feelings, and behaviours that stem from incongruence are forms of psychopathology. Thus, all of us are psychopathological, in some ways, at some times, to some greater or lesser extent. Psychopathology is not a categorical entity (i.e., present or absent), but rather a continuous one (i.e., present to some greater or lesser extent). As we shall go on to describe later, these views form the fundamental assumptions of what is now being referred to as 'positive clinical psychology' (Maddux et al., 2004b).

Normality versus abnormality

There have always been critics of a psychiatric establishment that makes judgement over normal versus abnormal behaviours. The difficulties in distinguishing 'normal' from 'abnormal' behaviour were highlighted in a classic study by Rosenhan (1973, 1975). Rosenhan conducted a now famous experiment in a real-life situation showing that psychiatrists' diagnoses were influenced by the social context.

Rosenhan's research team of eight 'normal' people visited 12 different mental hospitals saying that they were experiencing auditory hallucinations and hearing voices saying words like 'dull', 'thud', and 'empty'. This was part of the experiment. They were not really hearing voices, and they proceeded to answer all the other questions they were asked by the medical staff honestly. However, most of Rosenhan's team were admitted to hospital and diagnosed as schizophrenic. Once inside, the task of the research team (now pseudo-patients) was to convince the hospital staff that they were 'sane'. While inside the hospital the pseudo-patients behaved 'normally' and insisted on their 'sanity'. The pseudo-patients were hospitalised for between seven to 52 days with an average length of stay of 19 days. When discharged, the members of the research team were diagnosed as schizophrenic in remission. But what was most interesting was that while they were inside, their 'normal' behaviours were perceived by staff as indicating evidence of schizophrenia. Interestingly, however, some of the other patients were able to identify the pseudo-patients as impostors.

The next step in Rosenhan's research was perhaps even more interesting. Rosenhan informed psychiatric hospitals that pseudo-patients would again present themselves at the hospitals over the next few months. This time, however, there were no pseudo-patients. But, around one-fifth of patients admitted during this time were actually identified by staff as being pseudo-patients (Rosenhan, 1975). The studies by Rosenhan are often taken as evidence for how diagnosis is uncertain and can lead to labelling, and how once a label is attached to a person it becomes a self-fulfilling prophecy.

The experiment by Rosenhan raised important questions about who decides, and on what basis, what is 'normal' and what is 'abnormal'. Much work has accumulated telling us that considerations of what is 'normal' and what is 'abnormal' are not value free. Rather, considerations of 'normality' and 'abnormality' are bound up in cultural and historical contexts (see Littlewood & Lipsedge, 1993). For this reason, critics of the medical model of psychopathology have viewed diagnosis of people as suffering from psychiatric disorders as intrinsically harmful. Maslow summed this up in describing the use of words such as patient:

> I hate the medical model that they imply because the medical model suggests that the person who comes to the counsellor is a sick person, beset by disease and illness, seeking a cure. Actually, of course, we hope that the counsellor will be the one who helps to foster the self-actualisation of people, rather than the one who helps to cure a disease.
>
> (Maslow, 1993, p. 49)

Although there have been many previous critics of the medical model as a way of understanding psychopathology (see Sanders, 2005), many more researchers from within the new positive psychology movement are also now beginning to doubt the validity of the medical model for understanding psychological problems (see Hubble & Miller, 2004; Maddux, 2002; Maddux, Gosselin, & Winstead, 2004a; Maddux et al., 2004b; Yalom, 2001). Recently, in the letters page of the house journal of the British Psychological Society, *The Psychologist*, Marzillier (2004) wrote:

> I am interested in the truth. As a psychotherapist I am confronted every day by the knowledge that evidence-based psychotherapy is a myth. Yet all around me others are extolling its virtues. Do I remain silent because the truth is unpalatable? Or because it might lead to the underfunding of psychotherapy in the NHS [British National Health Service] or some other unwanted consequence? In his wise and useful book on psychotherapy Irvin Yalom pointed out that 'if we take the DSM diagnostic system too seriously, if we really believe we are carving at the joints of nature, then we may threaten the human, the spontaneous, the creative and uncertain nature of the therapeutic venture'. Psychotherapy is a creative and uncertain business. It should not be reduced to a collection of treatments for mythical illnesses.
>
> (Marzillier, 2004, pp. 625–626)

As an alternative to the medical model we have proposed the adoption of a conceptual model based on people's inherent tendency toward actualisation, as conceptualised within the person-centred psychology of Carl Rogers. This view of human nature represents a different paradigm to the medical model that underlies much of contemporary clinical and counselling psychology. From the positive psychological perspective, what is appealing about the person-centred model is that it offers a way of thinking about the human condition that is simultaneously concerned with (1) the development and alleviation of psychopathology, and (2) the development and facilitation of well-being.

Thus, positive therapy as we envisage it represents something of a sea change in mainstream psychological practice as it rejects the medical model orientation of viewing psychological problems in the same way as medical conditions, i.e., a series of discrete conditions each requiring a particular form of treatment. As we set out later, the paradigm of positive therapy is one very much reflected in movements toward what has become known as 'positive clinical psychology' (Maddux et al., 2004b).

Positive therapy and positive clinical psychology

In their groundbreaking critical analysis of the philosophical origins of clinical psychology, and their subsequent development of what they describe as an agenda for 'positive clinical psychology', Maddux et al. (2004b) argued that clinical psychology is defined by its illness ideology. The origins of this illness ideology – which permeates modern clinical psychology – can be traced back to the earliest origins of the discipline.

The first 'psychological clinic' in the United States was founded by Lightner Witmer at the University of Pennsylvania in 1886 (Reisman, 1991). This is believed to have marked the beginning of clinical psychology in the United States. However, Witmer and his colleagues worked primarily with children who had learning or school problems – not with 'patients' with 'mental disorders'. As such, they were more influenced by psychometric theory and its emphasis on measurement than they were by psychoanalytic theory and its emphasis on psychopathology and illness.

However, the mood of clinical psychology changed radically with Freud's momentous visit to Clark University in 1909. Largely from this point forward, clinical psychology and psychiatry came to be dominated by psychoanalytic theory with its emphasis on hidden intrapsychic processes and sexual and aggressive urges (Korchin, 1976). There were also other powerful situational factors that influenced the adoption of the illness ideology by clinical psychology at this time.

First, clinical psychology practitioner training typically occurred in psychiatric hospitals and clinics, where clinical psychologists worked primarily as psycho-diagnosticians under the direction of psychiatrists trained in medicine and psychoanalysis. This led clinical psychologists to adopt, uncritically, the methods and assumptions of their psychiatrist counterparts, who were themselves trained specifically in the medical model and the illness ideology (which may be entirely appropriate for physical disorders, but not, we would argue, for psychological disorders).

Second, the US Veterans Administration, established shortly after World War II, developed training centres and standards for clinical psychologists, but primarily within psychiatric settings that were steeped in biological and psychoanalytic models. Again, to reject the medical model and its attendant illness ideology would have been anathema to clinical psychologists of this period.

Third, in 1967, the founding of the United States National Institute of Mental Health (NIMH), despite its name, focused all its millions of research and practice dollars on treating mental illness, which irrevocably shaped the direction and practice of clinical psychologists. Again, to reject the medical model and the illness ideology implicit within it would have been to reject one's opportunity of this research and practice funding – a stiff test of theoretical values against pragmatic career choices.

Fourth, within the United Kingdom, clinical psychology was introduced under the auspices of Hans Eysenck at the Institute of Psychiatry following a tour of the United States and an examination of their clinical psychology training programmes (see Lavender, 2003). Within the UK itself, the climate at the Institute of Psychiatry was very informed by cognitive-behavioural approaches to therapy, and one that emphasised the 'scientist–practitioner' model. Thus, these concepts were implicitly enshrined within the British approach to clinical psychology and clinical psychology training, and were adopted, largely uncritically, from the predominant American model.

Fifth, the assumptions of clinical psychology, grounded in the illness ideology, were enshrined in the standards for clinical psychology training at the American Psychological Association

conference in Boulder, Colorado, in 1950. This led to 'the uncritical acceptance of the medical model, the organic explanation of
mental disorders, with psychiatric hegemony, medical concepts,
and language', and became the 'fatal flaw' of the scientist–
practitioner model that 'has distorted and damaged the development of clinical psychology ever since' (Albee, 2000, p. 247).

Grounded in this medico-psychiatric historical context, the
illness ideology has permeated the language of clinical psychology,
leading it to become the language of medicine and psychopathology. Characterised thus, clinical psychology narrows our focus to
what is weak and deficient rather than what is strong and healthy.
It emphasises abnormality over normality, poor adjustment over
healthy adjustment, and sickness over health.

Further, this illness ideology prescribes a certain way of thinking
about psychological problems, and further tells us what aspects of
human behaviour we should pay attention to. Maddux et al.
(2004a) identified three primary ways in which the uncritical
adoption of the illness ideology determined the remit and scope of
clinical psychology. First, it promotes dichotomies between normal
and abnormal behaviours, between clinical and non-clinical problems, and between clinical populations and non-clinical populations. Second, it locates human maladjustment inside the person,
rather than in the person's interactions with the environment and
their encounters with sociocultural values and social institutions.
Third, it portrays people who seek help as victims of intrapsychic
and biological forces beyond their control, and thus leaves them as
passive recipients of an expert's care.

As such, the medical model and illness ideology of clinical
psychology can be seen to be founded on four basic assumptions
(Maddux et al., 2004a):

- *Assumption 1*: clinical psychology would be concerned with
  psychopathology – deviant, abnormal and maladaptive behavioural and emotional conditions. Thus the focus was not on
  facilitating mental health but on alleviating mental illness.
  This excluded the millions of people who might experience
  problems in everyday living for the benefit of the much smaller
  number of people experiencing severe conditions.
- *Assumption 2*: psychopathology, clinical problems, and clinical populations, differ in *kind*, not just in degree, from normal
  problems in living, non-clinical problems and non-clinical

populations: they are considered to be independent and distinct entities. This *categorical model* presents the remit of clinical psychology as being categorically different to normal problems, thus requiring different theories.

- *Assumption 3*: psychological disorders are analogous to biological or medical diseases in that they reflect conditions inside the individual (the 'illness analogy'), rather than in the person's interactions with his or her environment.
- *Assumption 4*: following on from this illness analogy, the role of the clinical psychologist is to identify (diagnose) the disorder inside the person (patient) and to prescribe an intervention (treatment) for eliminating (curing) the internal disorder (disease). These interventions are referred to as *treatment* or *therapy*, unlike often equally successful attempts on the part of friends, family, teachers, and ministers.

However, positive psychological approaches to clinical psychology reject these implicit assumptions, as does the positive therapy approach, and instead present the assumptions of a positive clinical psychology (Maddux, et al., 2004a):

- *Assumption 1*: positive clinical psychology is concerned with everyday problems in living as much as it is with the more extreme variants of everyday functioning, that we might refer to as psychopathology. Positive clinical psychology is also as much concerned with understanding and enhancing subjective well-being and effective functioning as it is with alleviating subjective distress and maladaptive functioning.
- *Assumption 2*: psychopathology, clinical problems, and clinical populations, differ *only in degree*, rather than in kind, from normal problems in living, non-clinical problems and non-clinical populations: they are considered to be related entities falling somewhere on a *continuum* of human functioning. This *dimensional model* suggests a focus on health and fulfilment as much as on illness and distress, since they are related constructs that can be defined by the same psychological theories. Within this dimensional model, normality and abnormality, wellness and illness, and effective and ineffective psychological functioning lie along a *continuum* of human functioning. They are not separate and distinct entities, but are

rather considered as extreme variants of normal psychological phenomena.

- *Assumption 3*: psychological disorders are *not* analogous to biological or medical diseases. Rather, they are reflective of problems in the person's interactions with his or her environment, and not only and simply of problems within the person himself or herself. Further, these problems in living are not construed as being located within an individual, but rather are construed as being located within the interactions between an individual, other people, and the larger culture. This demands a closer inspection of the much more complex interplay of psychological, social and cultural factors that bear on an individual's psychological health.

- *Assumption 4*: following on from these three former assumptions, the role of the positive clinical psychologist is to identify human strengths and promote mental health as assets which buffer against weakness and mental illness. The people who seek this assistance are clients or students, not patients, and the professionals providing these approaches may be teachers, counsellors, consultants, coaches, or even social activists, and not just clinicians or doctors. The strategies and techniques they use are educational, relational, social, and political, not medical interventions. Further, the facilities providing this assistance may be centres, schools, or resorts, and not clinics or hospitals.

Our presentation of positive therapy shares the same fundamental assumptions presented in 'positive clinical psychology' (Maddux et al., 2004b). Notably, however, positive clinical psychology has not (yet) explicitly adopted the actualising tendency as a meta-theoretical perspective. Even so, consideration of the key assumptions of positive clinical psychology, as described earlier, reveals them to be entirely consistent with the fundamental assumptions of positive therapy. Taken together, positive therapy and positive clinical psychology provide a clear and powerful alternative to the medical model, and offer an integrative way forward for therapists who wish to work with their clients in positive therapeutic ways. As Maddux et al. (2004a, p. 332) conclude: 'The major change for clinical psychology, however, is not a matter of strategy and tactic, but a matter of vision and mission.'

Applicability of the positive psychology approach

What we have argued is that person-centred personality theory provides an account of psychopathology that provides an alternative to the medical model. We have also shown how this alternative perspective is captured not only by our positive therapy approach, but also by movements toward a positive clinical psychology (Maddux et al., 2004b). However, although it is our view that a much wider range of expressions of psychopathology can be understood through the lens of person-centred personality theory than are currently, we are aware that this is a controversial position with which many would disagree. Many psychiatrists would argue – perhaps not surprisingly because of their medical background – that certain psychological problems, such as schizophrenia, are caused by abnormal biological states. It is not that we would necessarily agree with them, but what we want to make clear is that we are not saying that all expressions of psychopathology will be best understood through person-centred personality theory, only that we think a much wider range of problems can be understood this way than currently are (see Joseph & Worsley, 2005a). We need to begin to open our eyes to this possibility and to see where the boundaries of the person-centred approach truly fall.

We are certainly open to the possibility that some experiences do represent abnormal and disordered workings of human physiology and cognitive functioning. For example, schizophrenia, bipolar disorders, temporal lobe epilepsy, and organic brain diseases may fall within this category. Also, there may be some psychological problems that are best treated with specific interventions. As Seligman and Peterson (2003) note, there may be some clear specific treatments for some specific disorders, such as applied tension for blood and injury phobia, cognitive therapy for panic, and exposure for obsessive-compulsive disorder (for a review, see Seligman, 1994). What we are saying is that we do need to determine carefully when psychological problems are best understood through the lens of the medical model. But we should not assume that all psychological problems fall under the spotlight of the medical model and require differential treatment with medical, cognitive, or neuropsychological interventions.

However, when it comes to the majority of forms of psychological suffering and distress, the key implications of our positive psychology approach are: (1) the task is facilitate the client's organismic valuing process, and (2) the goals of therapy do not begin and end with the goal of the client being symptom free, as seen through the lens of a DSM diagnosis. Rather, the positive therapist, working to facilitate the client's OVP, would adopt a model of psychopathology grounded in the assumption of an innate actualising tendency, and would work with the goal of the facilitation of well-being. This is because, as we have seen, when one adopts a continuum model based on the concept of congruence (i.e., we are more or less 'well') rather than a categorical medical model (i.e., we are either 'ill' or 'not ill'), the facilitation of well-being is synonymous with the alleviation of ill-being. Alleviating psychopathology and facilitating well-being is a unitary task. As Shlien said in a talk originally given in 1956:

> [I]f the skills developed in psychological counselling can release the constructive capacities of malfunctioning people so that they become healthier, this same help should be available to healthy people who are less than *fully* functioning. If we ever turn towards positive goals of health, we will care less about where the person begins, and more about how to achieve the desired endpoint of the positive goals.
>
> (Shlien, 2003b, p. 26)

Research

As psychological scientists we are interested in measurement. Sometimes we may be interested in measurement of phenomena based on diagnostic categories, for example, depression, anxiety, or posttraumatic stress. We may wish to conduct research to show that a particular therapy is effective for a particular so-called 'disorder'. There is plenty of such research going on, but as we have argued earlier, there are those who would criticise such research because of the doubtful validity of the DSM system on which the categories of disorder are based. However, others may argue that even if this is the case such research is necessary for those psychological therapies to maintain their foothold in an increasingly resource-competitive health service. We have come to value the ideas inherent in person-centred psychology, but we are aware that these ideas are out of fashion, and if they are to be taken seriously there needs to be supportive research evidence. It will benefit the person-centred movement to produce good quality research that shows that client-centred therapy is effective in the treatment of the various so-called psychiatric disorders. Indeed, as we have already discussed, the recent work by King et al. (2000) showing that client-centred therapy is as effective in the treatment of depression as cognitive behavioural therapy, has provided the evidence that has helped the person-centred movement begin to gain footholds within the British National Health Service.

Thus we have no criticism with the idea of research per se – in fact, quite the opposite, since as academic psychologists a large part of our time is spent conducting and reporting research. Seeking the truth is one of the highest goals we may hold as scientists, and it is this that after all is the idea behind research. What we choose to research, however, says something about us and our values. Research is never value free. We see nothing wrong in evidence-based practice, but what currently passes for evidence-based practice is, in our view, often misunderstood, misquoted, and misguided, and driven by political motivations rather than the search for truth.

Research is not confined to DSM-derived constructs. There are numerous other constructs derived from person-centred theory that can equally well form the basis of research, for example, locus of evaluation, congruence, authenticity, conditions of worth, can all be measured and their relationships to other variables tested statistically in exactly the same way researchers have tested constructs from the medical model. Similarly, self-determination theory, as we have seen, has already provided a wealth of evidence for autonomy, competence, relatedness, and their relation to well-being. The constructs we choose to investigate depend on our research question. For example, as we shall go on to describe in Chapter 7, we have proposed a new organismic valuing theory of posttraumatic stress disorder and adversarial growth. This is an exciting new theory because it brings the principles of positive psychology and the ideas of person-centred theory to the understanding of posttraumatic stress and growth following adversity. We are reluctant to talk about disorder, but we also recognise the need to work and write in a way that is accessible to people from a range of professional spectra, and our theory helps us to speak to medically minded clinicians who are interested in disorder, as well as to more traditional person-centred theorists and the new generation of positive psychologists. In this way, we strive to build bridges and forge integration across a wide range of professional perspectives and occupational groups.

Much work now remains to be done to test our theory empirically, which will involve bringing together measurement tools to assess posttraumatic stress, but also the concept of unconditional positive regard. We hypothesise that unconditional positive regard in a person's life prior to an event will serve as a protective factor against the development of posttraumatic stress, and serve to facilitate adversarial growth when present after an event. We shall go on to say more about this shortly, but for the moment the point is to illustrate that as psychological scientists we have a duty to conduct research to provide evidence in support of our assertions. Carl Rogers was known to say that the facts are always friendly, and by this he did not mean that research was to be used to justify ourselves and our opinions, but rather that we should go with what the data tell us, developing our theories in the light of our observations and findings, constantly checking what we think against the scientific evidence. That is what we strive to do, and why we are eager to promote the research agenda into positive psychology and positive therapies.

Measuring well-being

Positive psychology is still relatively new and although psychologists have many measurement tools at their disposal, most of these are solely concerned with aspects of psychopathology (e.g., Corcoran & Fischer, 2000). There are hundreds of tests available to measure constructs such as anxiety, depression, stress, and so on, but comparatively few measures available yet for those working from the positive psychology perspective (although Lopez & Snyder, 2003, is a positive psychological assessment volume that provides a recent exception). In particular, there are few measures available to help us understand therapeutic practice and well-being.

Depression–happiness

In order to address one measurement need of the applied positive psychologist and positive therapist, we have developed a short questionnaire to measure the continuum of depression–happiness, called the short depression–happiness scale (SDHS) (Joseph,

Table 6.1 The short depression–happiness scale (SDHS)

A number of statements that people have made to describe how they feel are given here. Read each one and tick the box which best describes how frequently you felt that way in the past seven days, including today. Some statements describe positive feelings and some describe negative feelings. You may have experienced both positive and negative feelings at different times during the past seven days.

	Never	Rarely	Some-times	Often
1 I felt dissatisfied with my life				
2 I felt happy				
3 I felt cheerless				
4 I felt pleased with the way I am				
5 I felt that life was enjoyable				
6 I felt that life was meaningless				

Scoring key
For items 2, 4, and 5, never = 0, rarely = 1, sometimes = 2, often = 3
For items 1, 3, and 6, never = 3, rarely = 2, sometimes = 1, often = 0

Using the scoring key, add scores on all six items to give a total score, with a possible range of 0 to 18. Higher scores indicate greater happiness. As scores decrease, happiness fades into unhappiness, which fades into depression. Research estimates that scores below 9 are increasingly indicative of depressive states.

Linley, Harwood, Lewis, & McCollam, 2004) (see Table 6.1). The SDHS is a six-item self-report questionnaire. Three items ask about positive thoughts, feelings, and bodily experiences. Three items ask about negative thoughts, feelings, and bodily experiences. Respondents are asked to think about how they have felt in the past seven days and to rate the frequency of each item on a four-point scale: *never* (0), *rarely* (1), *sometimes* (2), and *often* (3). Items concerning negative thoughts, feelings, and bodily experiences are reverse scored so that when all six items are summed respondents can potentially score between 0 and 18, with higher scores indicating greater frequency of positive thoughts and feelings and lower frequency of negative thoughts and feelings, happiness. The average score is around 12.

Through the zero point

Conceptually, the SDHS is similar to the well-known faces scale developed by Andrews and Withey (1976), which asks respondents to rate how they feel using seven schematic faces whose expressions range along a continuum from very negative (imagine a face with a down-turned mouth) to very positive (imagine a face with an up-turned mouth). Thus, the advantage of the SDHS over traditional self-report measures of depression (see Corcoran & Fischer, 2000) is that it not only allows us to assess the alleviation of depression, but also allows us to assess the extent to which the client is moving toward more happy and satisfied living. The SDHS allows the practitioner or researcher to assess change from states of depression to states of happiness, while avoiding the floor effects that might be encountered with well-used measures of depression such as the Beck depression inventory (BDI). Floor effects are so called because a score of 0 on the BDI, while indicative of the absence of depression, is not per se indicative of the presence of happiness. As such, the SDHS has the ability to avoid the floor effects that limit other measures of only depression, thus making it a potentially very useful measure for therapeutic practice.

To develop the questionnaire we went through extensive psychometric work to show that the scale has a single-factor structure, acceptable levels of internal consistency reliability, and convergent validity with other measures (see Joseph & Lewis, 1998; Joseph et al., 2004). We do not intend the word depression here to refer to a particular clinical state associated with a DSM diagnosis, but to a general reduced affect and loss of vitality, although for those interested in clinical use our preliminary research suggests that a score of 9 and below represents increasing risk of serious problems of depression. We would expect that the client group of most therapists will score in this region. But we would caution that we now need to subject the SDHS to further research in order to develop normative data.

We wanted a short questionnaire so that practitioners, as well as researchers, would be able to measure states of depression/happiness quickly and easily. This is important, particularly for practitioners, who may want clients to complete questionnaires as part of their own research and evaluation, and thus do not wish to burden their client with having to complete excessive questionnaires. The use of tests is a controversial topic as we have seen in

Chapter 5. Often, for research purposes in clinical settings, the therapist may want the client to complete questionnaires at regular intervals over the course of therapy, thus making it even more important that the questionnaire is short and easy to complete. The SDHS meets all these needs.

Thus, we think that the SDHS will be useful to practitioners and researchers who are in need of a short but reliable and valid measure of well-being. The SDHS is the only measure of which we are aware that provides clinicians with a rapid method of assessment with which to assess therapeutic change from states of depression through to states of happiness. There are now suggestions for various positive psychology interventions with clinical and health related populations, and the SDHS promises to provide a useful tool for researchers wishing to assess the effectiveness of their interventions.

Conclusion

As we have seen, positive psychology as we understand it rejects the categorical approach to psychopathology that is current within clinical psychology and the DSM (Maddux, 2002; Maddux et al., 2004b). An alternative is person-centred personality theory, which, as we have seen, accounts for both psychopathology and well-being through its premise that psychopathology stems from incongruence, i.e., the extent that people are not acting in accord with their OVP. Well-being arises to the extent that people are organismically valuing in their choices and behaviours. Further, we have shown that person-centred personality theory is also entirely consistent, if not fully synonymous, with the assumptions of positive clinical psychology, and which we have adopted within our understanding of positive therapy.

This integrative theory therefore provides a natural continuum that accounts for the varying extents of human experience of psychopathology and well-being, hence, the categorical distinction between positive and negative is viewed as inappropriate, since they are both part of the same vein of human experience. There is much debate by person-centred practitioners about the use of diagnosis and assessment, and one can understand this debate, given that their position is that there is no need for diagnosis, because there is no need to determine a specific treatment.

In summary, in talking about the ways we can work therapeutically to facilitate movement toward well-being, the impression may sometimes be given that positive therapy is just for the promotion of well-being, and would not be suitable for people with severe and chronic psychological problems. This is because the actualising tendency is an alternative paradigm to the medical model. Psychological problems are seen as resulting from the thwarting of the tendency towards actualisation, and the nature of each person's psychological problems can be understood when we know more about their developmental social–environmental conditions and the values and beliefs that they have internalised. The actualising tendency provides a holistic framework that simultaneously spans psychopathology and well-being. In facilitating the actualising tendency, the therapist is both alleviating psychopathology and promoting well-being. We are not saying that we need to reject the medical approach altogether when thinking about psychological problems: some psychopathology might be best considered as disorder, and treated within the medical field by psychiatrists and clinical psychologists. However, the idea that all psychological problems are best understood through the lens of the medical model and require specific treatments is an unfounded assumption, and one that we reject within positive therapy, and as we have shown, which is also rejected by positive psychologists more widely as they move towards a positive clinical psychology.

Chapter 7

Adaptation to threatening events: A positive psychology approach

Much of our own research programme has been concerned with how people respond to adversity. There is now much evidence that traumatic and stressful events can precipitate various psychological problems, including depression, anxiety, and symptoms of posttraumatic stress (Joseph, Williams, & Yule, 1995, 1997). However, more recently we have been developing a positive psychology approach to understanding stress and trauma. At first glance, the study of stressful and traumatic events might appear to be the nemesis of positive psychology. However, a number of philosophies, and literatures throughout human history have conveyed the idea that there is personal gain to be found in suffering (Linley, 2003). The observation that stressful and traumatic events can provoke positive psychological changes is also contained in the major religions of Buddhism, Christianity, Hinduism, Islam, and Judaism. Within humanistic and existential philosophy and psychology it has also long been recognised that positive changes can come about as a result of suffering (e.g., Frankl, 1963; Jaffe, 1985; Kessler, 1987).

The fact that stressful and traumatic events can provide opportunities for positive reappraisal and personal growth has also long been noted throughout the literatures on stress and coping (e.g., Antonovsky, 1987; Lazarus & Folkman, 1984; Taylor, 1983) and posttraumatic stress (e.g., Finkel, 1975; Herman, 1992; Janoff-Bulman, 1992; Joseph et al., 1997; Lyons, 1991; Snape, 1997). However, it is only relatively recently that the topic of growth through adversity has become the focus for much empirical and theoretical work (e.g., Joseph & Linley, 2005b; Linley & Joseph, 2004c; 2005; O'Leary & Ickovics, 1995; Tedeschi & Calhoun, 2004; Tedeschi, Park, & Calhoun, 1998a). In this chapter we will describe our own theoretical model of positive adversarial growth. The present chapter is an adaptation of work published previously (Joseph & Linley, 2005b) although here we have taken the opportunity to talk more about the therapeutic implications of our theory.

Growth following trauma and adversity

Growth through adversity seems to have three main facets. First, people often report that their relationships are enhanced in some way, for example that they now value their friends and family more, and feel an increased compassion and altruism toward others. Second, survivors change their views of themselves in some way, for example, that they have a greater sense of personal resiliency, wisdom, and strength, perhaps coupled with a greater acceptance of their vulnerabilities and limitations. Third, there are often reports of changes in life philosophy, for example, survivors report finding a fresh appreciation for each new day, and renegotiating what really matters to them in the full realisation that their life is finite (see Calhoun & Tedeschi, 1999; Linley, 2003; McMillen, 1999; Tedeschi, Park, & Calhoun, 1998b; Yalom, 1980; Yalom & Lieberman, 1991). For some, there is also a religious or spiritual component to their changes in life philosophy (Calhoun, Cann, Tedeschi, & McMillan, 2000: Koenig, Pargament, & Nielsen, 1998; Shaw, Joseph, & Linley, 2005).

These positive changes in psychological well-being can underpin a whole new way of living that embraces the central tenets of positive psychology (e.g., Linley, 2000, 2003; Seligman, 2003a). People may learn to appreciate each day to the full (i.e., positive subjective experience). They may believe themselves to be wiser or act more altruistically in the service of others (i.e., positive individual characteristics). They may dedicate their energies to social renewal or political activism (i.e., positive institutions and communities). There is a shift from the self-perception of oneself as a victim to that of a survivor. However, trauma survivors embrace this positive approach to life within a context of tragic hopefulness. They know firsthand the ups and downs, and the limits of human life. This awareness guides them to live their lives in a way that is truly and positively authentic, interpreting their trauma as a valued learning opportunity and giving back to others through the benefit of their experience.

Adversarial growth

We have introduced the new term 'adversarial growth' to describe the constellation of positive changes reported by people following stressful and traumatic events (Linley & Joseph, 2004d). Although we have employed the term adversarial growth, other authors have used terms such as construing benefits (Affleck & Tennen, 1996), perceived benefits (McMillen & Fisher, 1998), posttraumatic growth (Tedeschi & Calhoun, 1996), stress-related growth (Armeli, Gunthert, & Cohen, 2001; Park, 1998; Park, Cohen, & Murch, 1996), transformational coping (Aldwin, 1994), and thriving (Abraido-Lanza, Guier, & Colon, 1998), to describe the same phenomenon.

Sometimes we have used these terms too, but what we like about the term adversarial growth over and above these other terms is that it captures what we see as the essence of what this phenomenon is all about. As we shall go on to describe below, growth seems to occur when a person's experience is conflicting with their assumptions about themselves and the world. It is the conflict between experience of the world and our assumptions about the world that creates an adversarial tension, in which the person must either revise their assumptions of the world to fit their experience, or they must perceive their experience in such a way as to fit in with their assumptions. We propose that growth can occur when we revise our assumptions as a result of this adversarial tension, and we revise our expectations and assumptions about the self and the world in a positive way.

A second reason we like the term adversarial growth is that although it is often personally life-threatening and traumatic events that lead to growth, traumatic events are not necessary for growth to take place. But, other terms like posttraumatic growth can mislead people into thinking that growth can only occur after trauma. Further, since 'traumatic stress' is a specific disorder within the terms of the DSM, people have been led to think that for growth to occur, one must experience a 'trauma' as defined within the context of the DSM. But this is not so, since any experience that possesses the ability to create a conflict with assumptions about the self and the world can lead to growth. A sharp but truthful word from a friend or a colleague can challenge our self-perception, and lead to growth. Also, other terms like posttraumatic growth can be mistaken to imply that the person must first have a diagnosis of posttraumatic stress disorder before they can develop posttraumatic growth. For these reasons, we prefer to use the term adversarial growth.

Measurement of growth

The range of events that have been found to act as triggers to growth is wide. For example, positive changes of one sort or another have been reported following bereavement, accidents, disasters, illness, war and conflict, sexual assault, sexual abuse (see Linley & Joseph, 2004c; Tedeschi & Calhoun, 2004b, for recent reviews). A variety of measures have been developed to assess personal growth and positive change through adversity, and in our own research programme we have used the changes in outlook questionnaire (CiOQ) originally developed by Joseph, Williams, and Yule (1993) (see Table 7.1). The CiOQ provides a self-report assessment, in keeping with positive psychology, of the extent to which a person has experienced both positive changes and negative changes following adversity and trauma. The CiOQ consists of 26 items, 11 assess positive changes and 15 assess negative changes. The 11 positive items are summed to give a total score ranging from 11 to 66. The 15 negative items are summed to give a total score ranging from 15 to 90.

We have conducted extensive work into the psychometric properties of the CiOQ confirming its reliability and validity (see Joseph et al., 2005). We have also used it in a number of studies, documenting changes in people following, for example, the events of 9/11 (Linley et al., 2003) and in therapists who work with distressed people following trauma (Linley, Joseph, & Loumidis, 2005). In one study, it was used to assess positive changes in patients undergoing treatment for cancer. A large percentage of patients endorsed positive changes. The change that was most agreed with was that of valuing relationships much more now, followed by not taking life for granted any more (see Martin, Tolosa, & Joseph, 2004) (see Table 7.2).

The CiOQ promises to be a useful tool when working with clients who have experienced trauma and adversity. For practitioners who may need brief, and quick to administer, measures we have also developed a short version of the CiOQ (Joseph, Linley, Shevlin, Goodfellow, & Butler, 2006). The positive therapy approach involves a shift in perception from the medical

Table 7.1 Changes in outlook questionnaire (CiOQ)

Each of the following statements was made by people who experienced stressful and traumatic events in their lives about how the event had changed them. Thinking about how you have changed since the event, read each one and indicate, by circling the number, how much you agree or disagree with it *at the present time.*

	Strongly disagree	Disagree	Disagree a little	Agree a little	Agree	Strongly agree
1 I don't look forward to the future any more	1	2	3	4	5	6
2 My life has no meaning any more	1	2	3	4	5	6
3 I no longer feel able to cope with things	1	2	3	4	5	6
4 I don't take life for granted any more	1	2	3	4	5	6
5 I value my relationships much more now	1	2	3	4	5	6
6 I feel more experienced about life now	1	2	3	4	5	6
7 I don't worry about death at all any more	1	2	3	4	5	6
8 I live everyday to the full now	1	2	3	4	5	6
9 I fear death very much now	1	2	3	4	5	6
10 I look on each day as a bonus	1	2	3	4	5	6
11 I feel as if something bad is just around the corner waiting to happen	1	2	3	4	5	6
12 I'm a more understanding and tolerant person now	1	2	3	4	5	6
13 I have a greater faith in human nature now	1	2	3	4	5	6
14 I no longer take people or things for granted	1	2	3	4	5	6

continues overleaf

Table 7.1 Continued

	Strongly disagree	Disagree	Disagree a little	Agree a little	Agree	Strongly agree
15 I desperately wish I could turn the clock back to before it happened	1	2	3	4	5	6
16 I sometimes think it's not worth being a good person	1	2	3	4	5	6
17 I have very little trust in other people now	1	2	3	4	5	6
18 I feel very much as if I'm in limbo	1	2	3	4	5	6
19 I have very little trust in myself now	1	2	3	4	5	6
20 I feel harder towards other people	1	2	3	4	5	6
21 I am less tolerant of others now	1	2	3	4	5	6
22 I am much less able to communicate with other people	1	2	3	4	5	6
23 I value other people more now	1	2	3	4	5	6
24 I am more determined to succeed in life now	1	2	3	4	5	6
25 Nothing makes me happy any more	1	2	3	4	5	6
26 I feel as if I'm dead from the neck downwards	1	2	3	4	5	6

NB: Items 4, 5, 6, 7, 8, 10, 12, 13, 14, 23, and 24 are summated to give a total score for the positive response scale (CiOP). Items 1, 2, 3, 9, 11, 15, 16, 17, 18, 19, 20, 21, 22, 25, and 26 are summated to give a total score for the negative response scale (CiON).

Table 7.2 Percentage of respondents (n = 76) following cancer treatment agreeing with each of the statements on the CiOQ positive scale

	% strongly agreed	% agreed	% agreed a little
I value my relationships much more now	53	35	9
I don't take life for granted any more	47	39	8
I feel more experienced about life now	39	38	18
I no longer take people or things for granted	37	39	16
I live every day to the full now	36	41	14
I look on each day as a bonus	45	26	17
I value other people more now	32	41	15
I am more determined to succeed in life now	37	25	21
I'm a more understanding and tolerant person now	18	26	30
I have greater faith in human nature now	12	23	36
I don't worry about death at all any more	18	12	23

Source: Martin et al., 2004

model to the person-centred model, in which we begin to understand that the normal outcome of traumatic stress is growth rather than psychopathology. In the following section, we will describe how person-centred theory can be developed to understand response to traumatic events.

Organismic valuing and growth following adversity

Although the study of adversarial growth is relatively recent, as we have seen in Chapter 3, the characteristics of growth described earlier have long been of interest to humanistic psychologists. What we now call adversarial growth might be viewed in terms of a movement toward becoming what Rogers (1959) referred to as fully functioning (see Joseph, 2003b, 2004, 2005). As we discussed in Chapter 3, the fully functioning person is someone who is accepting of themselves; values all aspects of themselves – their strengths and their weaknesses; is able to live fully in the present; experiences life as a process; finds purpose and meaning in life; desires authenticity in themselves, others, and societal organisations; values deep trusting relationships; is compassionate toward others, and able to receive compassion from others; and is acceptant that change is necessary and inevitable. The characteristics of the fully functioning person are synonymous with those of adversarial growth. As with descriptions of adversarial growth, the description of the fully functioning person is primarily a description of the development of psychological well-being rather than subjective well-being (see also Chapter 2).

As we have seen, what Rogers (1959) proposed was that individuals have an innate tendency towards actualisation of their potentialities, and when individuals are provided with a facilitative social environment they will actualise towards becoming fully functioning people. In the person-centred psychology of Carl Rogers, the social environment necessary to facilitate this innate tendency towards actualisation is one characterized by unconditional positive regard. In brief, Rogers hypothesised that in an unconditionally positively regarding social environment, people drop their psychological defences so that they are able to realistically appraise the person–environment interaction. Through realistic appraisal processes, people are able to move psychologically towards becoming fully functioning. As we saw in Chapter 3, evidence suggests that people grow when there is contact with the organismic valuing process. We argue that individuals have innate developmental trends and propensities towards growth that may be given voice by an organismic valuing process occurring within them. A person-centred perspective on trauma emphasises that growth is the natural endpoint of trauma resolution (Joseph, 2003b, 2004, 2005; see also Christopher, 2004).

Shattered assumptions

The confrontation with an adverse event has a shattering effect on the person's assumptive world. Traumatic events show us that we are fragile, that the future is uncertain, and that life is not just. Traumatic events show us the limits of the human condition and bring into question our assumptions about ourselves and the world (Janoff-Bulman, 1989, 1992). The phenomenology of posttraumatic stress disorder (PTSD), the states of intrusion and avoidance, according to Horowitz (1982, 1986) and Janoff-Bulman (1992) are indicative of the need to cognitively and emotionally process the new trauma-related information and to rebuild a new assumptive world. As Creamer, Burgess, and Pattison (1992) argue, the symptoms of PTSD are indicative of network resolution processing, and the fact that the person is cognitively engaged in trying to work through their experience. Individual differences in trauma response are explained in organismic valuing process theory in terms of the degree of disparity between the trauma and pre-existing expectations and beliefs. Here is the notion that it is how a person perceives the event that is important.

Recovery from trauma in these theoretical perspectives is explained as resulting from either assimilation of the traumatic memory or a revision of existing schemas to cognitively accommodate new information. Organismic valuing process theory holds that it is human nature to rebuild a new assumptive world that positively accommodates the new trauma-related information. That is to say, people are intrinsically motivated to find meaning and seek benefit in their experience and the natural endpoint of trauma resolution is growth. But this does not always happen, unless the social environment provides the basic nutrients for growth (see Chapter 3).

Accommodation versus assimilation

Thus, our organismic theory posits that human beings are active, growth-oriented organisms. They are naturally inclined to cognitively accommodate their psychological experiences into a unified sense of self, and realistic view of the world. The process of cognitive accommodation is such that the person's assumptive world is rebuilt in the light of their experiences. This is in contrast to the process of cognitive assimilation where the person appraises their experiences in such a way as to be consistent with their assumptive world. Growth, by definition, requires accommodation rather than assimilation. However, although the theory says that people are intrinsically motivated toward accommodation, the theory also posits that extrinsic social–environmental forces can usurp this process leading the person to assimilate rather than accommodate. For example, within the social psychology literature there is much work on how victims will often self-blame inappropriately in order to maintain their sense of the world as just and controllable (see Joseph, 1999). If an event happens which seems to be for no reason this can be unsettling, and so people sometimes cope with such events by perceiving themselves as to blame, which although providing an explanation for what happened that is more settling, is obviously unhelpful in other ways.

How we make sense of the world around us is, of course, influenced by the people around us. Other people influence our appraisal processes, and can therefore say and do things that will either facilitate or impede the process of accommodation. In the last example, perhaps others are unsettled too, and in their attempts to be supportive inadvertently encourage us to self-blame, impeding the process of accommodation, and leading us to assimilate our experience. If we were to accommodate our experience, we would rebuild our worldview to acknowledge that events are sometimes random and strike us for no good reason. This might be unsettling but it is true. To assimilate the experience means to defend ourselves from this truth.

Meaning as comprehension versus meaning as significance

Thus, the organismic valuing theory of growth through adversity posits an intrinsic motivation toward cognitive accommodation of the new trauma-related information. Accommodation requires a shift in meaning, of which two kinds can be delineated, a shift in meaning as comprehension, and shift in meaning as significance (e.g., Davis, Nolen-Hoeksema, & Larson, 1998; Janoff-Bulman & McPherson Frantz, 1997). Cognitive accommodation processes require changes in meaning as significance, and this can be in either a negative or a positive direction. A person can accommodate new trauma-related information, for example, that random events happen in the world and that bad things can happen at any time, in one of two ways. This accommodation may be made in a negative direction (e.g., a depressogenic reaction of hopelessness and helplessness), or in a positive direction of meaning as significance (e.g., that life is to be lived more in the here and now). It is thought that it is human nature to be intrinsically motivated towards a positive accommodation of the new trauma-related information as opposed to a negative accommodation, insofar as an evolutionary psychology approach would suggest that this should be more adaptive. As Christopher (2004) more recently points out, in describing a theory that extensively fills out the biological aspects of reactions to trauma, from an evolutionary point of view trauma breaks up culturally acquired attitudes and creates the possibility of new meanings and more adaptive responses to the environment.

Three cognitive outcomes

In this theory, the states of intrusion and avoidance characteristic of PTSD are indicative of cognitive-emotional processing and the need to rebuild the assumptive world. Thus, PTSD will diminish to the extent that the new trauma-related information is either accommodated or assimilated. As the person begins to either accommodate or assimilate their experience, there are three possible endpoints.

Three cognitive outcomes to the psychological resolution of trauma-related difficulties are therefore posited. First, that experiences can be assimilated (i.e., return to pre-trauma baseline), second, that experiences can be accommodated in a negative direction (i.e., psychopathology), and third, that experiences can be accommodated in a positive direction (i.e., growth). As an analogy, imagine a person is picking up the pieces of a shattered vase. He or she can attempt to put the vase back together exactly as it was (assimilation), but now the vase is more fragile, covered in fractures and held together with sticking tape. Alternatively, the pieces can be discarded and placed in the trash (negative accommodation) or used to build something new, perhaps part of a beautiful mosaic (positive accommodation).

The possibility of the three cognitive outcomes helps to resolve the question of why it is that previously traumatised people often appear to be more vulnerable rather than more resistant to the effects of future stressful and traumatic events. We expect that attempts at assimilation rather than accommodation are most common in practice. People who assimilate their experience thus maintain their pre-event assumptions despite the evidence to the contrary, and thus would be expected to develop more rigid defences, which in turn leaves them at increased vulnerability for future development of posttraumatic stress.

In summary, what the organismic valuing process theory posits is that the person is intrinsically motivated toward the rebuilding of an assumptive world in a direction consistent with the new trauma-related information. This leads to greater psychological well-being, although not necessarily greater subjective well-being. The theory holds that this occurs when the social environment is able to meet the individual's needs for autonomy, competence, and relatedness, then the organismic valuing process is promoted. An organismic valuing theory of adversarial growth is therefore consistent with and able to integrate the theoretical themes discussed earlier. First, organismic valuing process theory is first and foremost a theory of psychological well-being. Second, organismic valuing process theory is consistent with the notion of an underlying completion principle, but extends this concept so that the completion principle is viewed as an expression of part of the tendency towards actualisation. Third, organismic valuing theory is consistent with the notion that accommodation rather than assimilation is necessary for growth. Fourth, organismic valuing process theory is consistent with the notion that it is meaning as significance that underlies growth rather than meaning as comprehensibility.

What the organismic valuing process theory posits is that the person is intrinsically motivated toward the rebuilding of the assumptive world in a direction consistent with their innate propensities toward actualisation of the potentialities. As part of this innate process the individual is motivated to engage in a realistic reappraisal of the meaning of the event and its existential implications. This leads to greater psychological well-being. For most we expect that the adversarial growth is a process that unfolds gradually over a period of time as the person cognitively accommodates the new trauma-related material, and appraises the meaning significance of the accommodation.

Facilitating growth after adversity

From an applied perspective, clinicians should be aware of the potential for positive change in their clients following trauma and adversity. Positive changes may be used as foundations for further therapeutic work, providing hope that the trauma can be overcome (Calhoun & Tedeschi, 1999; Linley & Joseph, 2002a; Tedeschi & Calhoun, 2004). Interventions for posttraumatic stress disorder typically do not take account of the potential for adversarial growth, and Calhoun and Tedeschi (1999) caution that approaches to interventions that aim to help the client can inadvertently serve to stifle the possibility of growth. Essentially, all trauma theorists are in agreement that recovery involves some form of cognitive restructuring (Foa & Kozak, 1986; Foa & Rothbaum, 1998). The terms assimilation and accommodation have been used but not always in the systematic theoretical way we have employed them. Our hypothesis is that the alleviation of posttraumatic stress may come about through either assimilation or accommodation processes, but only accommodation can be growthful. But accommodation is in itself not necessarily growth-ful, as the new trauma-related information can be accommodated either negatively or positively. What determines the direction of accommodation is the extent to which the person is able to organismically evaluate their experiences.

Organismic valuing process theory suggests that what is paramount in facilitating growth after adversity is helping the client to hear their own inner voice of wisdom and to articulate their own inner experiencing, and thus to accommodate the new trauma-related information rather than assimilate it. As Roth, Lebowitz, & DeRosa (1997) write:

> Researchers and clinicians evaluating traumatic meanings must access the wise and adaptive part of the victim's mind that is holding the trauma in anticipation of finding a place for it to rest in peace.
>
> (Roth, Lebowitz, & DeRosa, 1997, p. 515)

The implication of organismic valuing process theory is that, depending on the therapist's fundamental assumptions and way of working, they could help the client to either assimilate or accom-modate the new trauma-related information. The theory suggests that a therapist who listens attentively and actively to the client, and helps the client to more clearly articulate the client's own new meanings as they begin to emerge, will be helping to facilitate the organismic valuing process, and thus to accommodate the new trauma-related information in a positive direction. In contrast, a therapist whose style of working more reflects their own values or other social conventions might serve to facilitate the client's accommodation process in either a negative or positive direction, depending on those values and conventions and the extent to which they are congruent with the client's organismic valuing.

Alternatively, we might reassure someone in such a way as to foster the process of assimilation. For example, events in which self-esteem comes under threat, people will be motivated to blame others in order to maintain their self-esteem. For events in which the sense of the just world is under threat, people will be moti-vated to blame themselves to maintain their sense of justice. These are the costs and benefits of blame and how blaming can be used to help assimilate the new trauma-related information (Joseph, 1999).

Thus, a therapist may have the best intentions to help his or her client, but our theory suggests that unless the therapist is working within the client's frame of reference and taking care to facilitate the client's own articulation of meaning they could inadvertently be leading the client to assimilate or even negatively accommodate the new trauma-related information. In terms of the traditional concerns of clinical psychology, i.e., alleviating the so-called symptoms of PTSD, assimilation or negative accommodation might equally well lead to a reduction in symptoms, but they will not lead to growth. Growth, by definition, requires the positive accommodation of trauma-related information. Furthermore, although by indices of PTSD the outcome of either assimilation or negative accommodation might appear satisfactory, neither is a satisfactory outcome when looked at more broadly. Negative accommodation results in a new manifestation of psychopathology. Depending on the idiosyncratic nature of the person's cognitive accommodation, this could lead to feelings of anger, hostility, guilt, or shame, for example. Similarly, although assimilation processes may result in the reduction of PTSD as defined in DSM, it may be expected to result in a more fragile person, now more prone to future retraumatisation. Future research is now needed to test these predictions.

Following on from this academic research, we have begun to take an interest in the facilitation of adversarial growth, using person-centred methods as a means of facilitating our clients' organismic valuing processes (Joseph, 2004). For example, serious illness is often a trigger for growth, and the application of positive therapy to health psychology seems particularly relevant, particularly within the context of life threatening illness, such as cancer. As Yalom writes:

> A real confrontation with death usually causes one to question with real seriousness the goals and conduct of one's life up to then. So also with those who confront death through a fatal illness. How many people have lamented: 'what a pity I had to wait till now, when my body is riddled with cancer, to know how to live!'
>
> (Yalom, 1989, p. 26)

In England, one in three people will be diagnosed with cancer during their lifetime (Department of Health, 2000), and so helping people to live as fully as possible afterwards is an important goal for health psychology. In line with our views on facilitating the OVP, preliminary work was conducted to assess the experiences of cancer patients who were currently clear of their disease in person-centred groups. The work was carried out by a trainee clinical psychologist, Joanne Martin, in England under the supervision of Stephen Joseph and Inigo Tolosa, based at the Birmingham Cancer Centre (Martin, 2004). Eight people participated in the group, four men and four women ranging in age from 31 to 65 years. The women had all had diagnoses of breast cancer, the men either testicular cancer, lung cancer or lymphoma. Years since diagnosis ranged from one to five years. The groups ran for eight sessions, for 90 minutes, and were held twice weekly. Sessions were facilitated by Joanne who worked in a person-centred way, such that the group was client led.

Interviews were conducted with the participants one month after the end of the groups, and thematic analysis of the interview transcripts was conducted. Generally, participants were positive about their experiences. The most frequent theme was the opportunity to share experiences, to be understood, and to not feel alone in the experience:

> It was good that we could just talk freely, because I think we all just sort of found that outside whilst there can be people within your family, within your friends, who are around you, they themselves will have their own attitudes and some don't necessarily encourage you to speak about your own actual feelings, so that was good.
>
> Well, we were all in the same boat . . . and others don't understand.
>
> I think some of the things that go round in your head, you realise you're not the only one, you do realise that others have the same thoughts and feelings.

These preliminary pilot data are encouraging and point to a new line of research for the future. However, at present, we must recognise that as is so often the case, person-centred approaches to therapy, including that for people suffering the effects of traumatic

exposure, have not been investigated. Various cognitive-behavioural techniques have, however, been subject to empirical tests
and are recommended as the treatments of choice for PTSD (see,
for example, Foa, Keane, & Friedman, 2000). However, we would
caution that when it comes to understanding positive growth
processes we cannot just assume that what we know about the
alleviation of PTSD applies to the facilitation of growth. Furthermore, there is a need to understand all therapeutic work in relation
to the process of accommodation and assimilation, in the light of
our theoretical perspective that traditional treatments while helping to alleviate PTSD could possibly be unhelpful in other ways.

Conclusion

In this chapter, we have presented a new theory of how people
adapt, both positively and negatively, following exposure to
threatening and traumatic events. The organismic valuing theory
of growth through adversity draws from our own published work
(e.g., Joseph & Linley, 2005b), and provides a person-centred
account of adaptation to trauma that is an early example of the
positive therapy approach in practice. In essence, this theory pro-
poses that when people's basic psychological needs for autonomy,
competence, and relatedness are met through a supportive social
environment, then their organismic valuing process will be facilitated, and they will be able to accommodate positively the new
trauma material, changing their views and perceptions on account
of this new information. This positive accommodation leads to
increases in psychological well-being, but not necessarily increases
in subjective well-being, as the person rebuilds their assumptive
world in a way that is more congruent with their organismic
valuing process. These increases in psychological well-being are
characterised as adversarial growth, and also represent a movement towards becoming more fully functioning.

A fundamental element of this process is the role of the therapist, since the OVP theory of growth posits that the therapist
should only work to facilitate the OVP of the client, and should
not allow the therapy to be driven by the therapist's own agenda,
values, or beliefs. The danger of the therapist leading the therapy
encounter is that the client could be led to either assimilate the
trauma material, thus leaving them vulnerable in the future, or
negatively accommodate the trauma material, thus leaving them in

a state of incongruence. Our positive therapy approach, exemplified in the organismic valuing theory of growth through adversity, shows how this can come about. Finally in this chapter, we briefly described some early work that demonstrates the person-centred facilitation of adversarial growth in people following cancer, and we called for further research to test and elaborate the various aspects of both the organismic valuing theory of growth and the principles of positive therapy more broadly.

In the next chapter, we paint the canvas much more broadly, and go on to consider the social and political implications of the positive therapy approach, as well as addressing some of the issues of the sociocultural context of our work, and the need to be openly reflective about our therapeutic and professional practice.

Chapter 8

Conclusions: Reflections, context, and future

In this chapter we will explore in more detail some of the ideas mentioned briefly earlier, in particular the social and political considerations that arise out of our positive therapy approach. The first of these is the question of whose agenda do we, therapists, work to? Our answer to this depends on our deep-seated philosophical assumptions about human nature and the purpose of therapy. As we have seen, the therapy world can be divided into those who adopt the medical model, and those who favour humanistic and social constructivist approaches (O'Hara, 1997).

As psychologists, we advocate therapeutic practice that is evidence based (Milne, 1999), and further research is needed to investigate the positive therapies. Our approach to positive therapy is based on the fundamental assumption that the client is their own best expert and that the role of the therapist is to facilitate the client in listening more attentively to their own inner voice, and to learn how to evaluate their experiences from an internal locus rather than an external locus. This approach has a lineage to the person-centred approach of Carl Rogers, and we propose the actualising tendency as the foundation of the positive therapies, with client-centred therapy being a quintessential positive therapy. The essence of client-centred therapy is the belief in the self-determination of the client, thus the therapist is non-directive (Levitt, 2005b). As we have seen throughout this book, whether one adopts this approach themselves comes down in the end to personal beliefs and fundamental assumptions about human nature. As Schmid (2005) wrote:

> Non-directivity is thus a matter of basic beliefs. People who think that directivity is necessary in therapy and counselling

have a different image of the human being, a different concept of how to deal with knowledge and a different ethical stance from those who work with their clients on the basis of non-directiveness. Since it is of no use to argue over beliefs (they precede acting, thinking, and science), there is no way to say who, ultimately, is right.

(Schmid, 2005, p. 82)

Client-centred therapy is an approach that stands in contrast to the medical model. For this reason, there is relatively limited research compared to other therapies showing it to be an effective way of working for the range of so-called psychiatric disorders as listed in the DSM. But, we have emphasised that this is only a valid criticism from the perspective of those who accept the medical model as the way to conceptualise psychological problems. As we have seen, client-centred therapists (e.g., Sanders, 2005) are now among a growing number of positive psychologists who also question the reliance of psychology on the medical model (see Maddux, 2002; Maddux et al., 2004a). As we have seen, as an alternative to the medical model, client-centred theorists adopt the alternative paradigm of the actualising tendency and how it becomes usurped by conditions of worth.

Personal transformation versus social adjustment

As we have seen in the previous chapters, the role of the positive therapist, as we have described him or her, is to help the client to hear their own inner voice. We recognise that there are other positive psychologists who may have different views on therapy to us, so we would emphasise that it is positive therapy, as we have envisaged it, that places emphasis on the organismic valuing process of the client. We also fully recognise that what we have to say here is not an established position among positive psychologists. As we have detailed throughout this book, theory suggests that the facilitation of the organismic valuing process leads to personal change in the direction of greater psychological well-being (e.g., autonomy, meaning, purpose, coherence, relatedness, etc.), which in turn leads to greater subjective well-being (greater happiness, less depression, increased life satisfaction, etc.). What makes positive therapy different is that it is concerned with personal transformation, and personal transformation is ultimately political. Personal transformation is political because it is about the person moving forward in their life, more consciously aware of their choices, and choosing their own path, rather than a path that has been prescribed by someone else. When that path becomes difficult the causes of the difficulty can be located within the social context rather than within the person.

Such personal change however is often at odds with the goals of professional psychologists whose agenda is not one of person transformation, but one of social adjustment. Many of the problems people have in living are a result of social forces, such as poor housing, unrewarding employment, financial difficulties, poor parenting, lack of education, emotional illiteracy, and so on. The evidence for this is overwhelming, since for over 40 years there has been a steady stream of research documenting the effects of negative life events, and the psychological effects of adverse social conditions (Hagan & Smail, 1997a, 1997b; Smail, 2005). Certainly, psychologists and psychiatrists will introduce social factors into their formulation and understanding of the client's problem, and in some cases will serve as advocates for their client in relation to social services or some other external agency. However, mostly psychologists and psychiatrists work at the level of the individual, either through therapy or drug administration, and it is the individual's cognitions, feelings, and behaviours, that are targeted in trying to help the person, not their social conditions. In this way, the 'problem' is located within the person, rather than within the person's interactions with their environment (cf. Maddux et al., 2004a, 2004b).

In so doing, the question we ask is to what extent the professions of psychology and psychiatry act as agents of social control helping people to adjust to their adverse living conditions, and thus serving to maintain social inequalities and injustices (see Proctor, 2005). Most psychologists and psychiatrists probably do not think of themselves in this way, which is, of course, how, critics of those professions say, they maintain their role as oppressive forces. This is not to say that these individuals or the professions as a whole deliberately set out to be forces of social control, but by adopting the medical model and viewing psychopathology as resulting from within the person as opposed to social context factors, this is inevitably what results. Of course, the same might be said for many counsellors and psychotherapists as well. As the existential therapist Rollo May described: 'Psychotherapists become the agents of the culture whose particular task it is to adjust people to it: psychotherapy becomes an expression of the fragmentation of the period rather than an enterprise for overcoming it' (May, 1994, p. 87). By the same token, there are many therapists, from all professions, who are well aware of these issues and who do strive to politicise therapy, and to make it clear just how important social environmental pressures are in the development of human distress (e.g., Hagan & Smail, 1997a, 1997b; Sanders, 2005; Smail, 1996, 2005).

Politicising therapy

For too long we think the profession of psychology and psychiatry, in particular, have attempted to maintain a politically neutral stance, with of course some notable exceptions (see Joseph, 2001, for a review). In looking back in particular to the ideas of Carl Rogers, we are aware that at the time of his writing about personal freedom and responsibility it was the era of McCarthyism in the United States. Although we would not claim we have returned to those days, perhaps our culture has changed over the last decade in ways that have diminished our freedom and increased our pressure to conform, in such a way that the person-centred approach again stands out more clearly against its cultural backcloth, with its emphasis on relationships, genuineness, and respect.

But now that these questions are being raised we can see that it is not possible to be politically neutral, all actions are value based and all behaviours must be dictated by some agenda. When we step into someone else's life to provide help on how to live that life, we are entering into the world of morality and politics. We can tell ourselves that we have no political ideology, but that does not mean we have *no* ideology. Furthermore, it is likely the denial of ideology is damaging to clients (Kearney, 1996). A recent exchange of letters in *The Psychologist*, the house journal of the British Psychological Society, raised some of these issues. In response to one letter, in which the author stated that she did not want to belong to a professional body that became involved with politics, Kidner (2001) wrote:

Whether we like it or not, psychology, like any discipline, contains an implicit political ideology: and silence or denial of our involvement is no less a political act than explicit political action. In the former case, however, our involvement takes the form of unconscious complicity in these social practices that we try to ignore. Ulfried Geuter (1992), in his thorough analysis of the growth of psychology in Nazi Germany, notes that 'in the course of the professionalisation of psychology . . . [psychologists] were relatively blind to, when they did not actively affirm, the social and political context in which professionalism took place'. . . . Moreover, 'the things that benefited the discipline or the profession were seen by many as being wholly good, no matter . . . in whose service' (p. 260). The choice we have to make, therefore, is not between involvement or non-involvement, but between awareness of our involvement or denial. As Geuter remarks: 'if the application of psychology is seen as neutral or even humane in principle, an absolute loyalty to the state has already worked its way into the self-image of the science.'

(Kidner, 2001, p. 178)

Our aims here are to emphasise that the practice of psychology and therapy is always political, and to provide a forum for greater professional self-reflection. As we have seen, we would argue that by our definition, positive therapy is about personal transformation and not social adjustment, because, as we have defined it, the foundation stone is that it is driven by the assumption that our task is to help clients to hear their own inner voice more clearly. In contrast, we believe that much of mainstream professional psychology is not about helping people to hear their own inner voice more clearly, but about facilitating change according to some externally driven agenda. We are not suggesting that psychologists who do this, do so intentionally, in the knowledge that they are serving to maintain a political status quo and are thwarting their client's potential for growth. After all, they are not working from within the person-centred model that provides this alternative viewpoint, but rather working from within the medical model that justifies their behaviour as being appropriate and helpful to the client.

That said, we do not see it as our role to provide an answer to the question of whose agenda professional psychologists ought to be working to. Perhaps it should be decided that the role of the psychologist is to be an agent of social control. What we are saying is that the question should not be ignored, but should be addressed. If the agenda of professional psychology is made explicit, then it is open to consideration, criticism and revision.

More cynically, to the extent that the agenda of the broader context is congruent with OVP of the person, the more likely it is to be successful. Consider, for example, that people satisfied at work are more productive (Judge, Thoresen, Bono, & Patton, 2001), that people who use their strengths and talents in the workplace make higher profits for their organisation (Hodges & Clifton, 2004), and that executive coaching is most effective when it harnesses the inner resources of the client (Kauffman & Scoular, 2004). Recognising the needs and aspirations of offenders, and facilitating them in finding legitimate ways to meet these needs and aspirations, leads to lower rates of reoffending (Ward & Mann, 2004). Health strategies are only effective if they serve the needs of the target population to at least a minimal extent (Huppert, 2004; Taylor & Sherman, 2004). Governments (at least in democratic societies) only remain in power if their policies are judged effective and appropriate by the voting public (Myers, 2004). Hence, the overall message is that if the agenda for practice is not the agenda of the individuals it is intended to target, it is far less likely to succeed than if it is congruent with the agenda of those individuals.

However, it is only in the most superficial way that the agenda of the factory worker, for example, can ever coincide with that of the factory owner. Thus, despite these examples, there is no shortage of employment for psychologists, which serves to illustrate the opposite use of psychology, and some obvious examples too – employment of commercial psychologists to help understand consumer behaviour related to cigarettes, gambling, shopping habits, with the goal of providing information that will increase cigarette consumption, gambling, and lead to increased materialism.

In turning our attention to the political agenda behind the practice of therapy, we are aware that similar ideas have been previously expressed by others. Jung talked of how the process of individuation leads eventually to the improvement of society (Donlevy, 1996). Rogers (1978) talked of the *quiet revolution* to describe the political agenda of how personal change leads to social change. As people change toward becoming more fully functioning, become more aware of their choices in life, and choose to pursue a life dictated by their own values, they will, according to Rogers, move toward becoming more socially constructive in their behaviour, thus more active politically, more open to the suffering of others, and more willing to engage at the social and political level.

Culture and materialism

In his book *To Have or To Be*, Fromm (1976) argued that the more fulfilling life was to be had through 'being' as opposed to 'having'. In particular, in this context we think the ideas we are expressing here from within the positive psychology movement, most echo those of Fromm (1976). His powerful writings on the nature of society show how the materialistic attitude has been detrimental to human welfare (see also Kasser, 2002). Fromm's writings suggested that the more fulfilling life was to be achieved through an acceptant attitude and an ability to be present and appreciative, something that is now receiving overwhelming support from the positive psychology research literature (Brown & Ryan, 2004; Kasser, 2004).

More recent writers have distinguished between terminal materialism (i.e., consumption of objects that is an end in itself) as opposed to instrumental materialism (i.e., possession of objects as the means for furthering personal and social goals) (Csikszentmihalyi & Rochberg-Halton, 1981). Whereas instrumental materialism is related to intrinsic motivation and is meaningful and leads to well-being, terminal materialism is damaging (see Kasser, 2002, 2004).

The use of these examples highlights our own cultural embeddedness and we would stress that positive psychology research findings, at least as developed within a Western liberal individualistic context, are not prototypically 'exportable' to countries or cultures that do not share our modern cultural identity. This should not be taken as a criticism, but rather as an open and reflective stance on the limits and scope of our positive psychology perspective.

Indeed, recognising our inevitable cultural embeddedness is the basis on which a full understanding of positive psychology rests. In being aware of these limits, we are able to be more fully respectful and tolerant of different traditions and approaches, especially in the recognition that we have as much to learn from them as they have from us. In terms of practice, these issues are fundamental as positive psychology seeks to extend its foundations further into

Europe and Asia, and also in being mindful of the practice of positive psychology in diverse multicultural settings within our own societies (cf. Eisenberg & Ota Wang, 2003; Lopez, Prosser, Edwards, Magyar-Moe, Neufeld, & Rasmussen, 2002).

What this serves to illustrate is that the value assumption of positive psychology, i.e., that the 'positive' is good, is itself culturally defined (cf. Christopher, 2003). As we have seen, Seligman and Csikszentmihalyi (2000) propose three levels of positive psychology: positive subjective experiences; positive individual characteristics; and positive institutions. But what are the value positions that underpin these three levels of the 'positive'? First, and as demonstrated by Christopher (1999), many Western values are implicitly imbued with the liberal individualism that characterises the current Western cultural and historical epoch. Thus, the Western way of understanding the world thinks primarily in terms of the individual as distinct from his or her community, culture, and cosmos, a view that is very different to many non-Western cultures (Shweder & Bourne, 1984). Second, Western society places greater emphasis on extrinsic values than intrinsic values. We grow up internalising values about how to lead our lives and what values to hold. Most of us in Western society will have grown up internalising values about the importance of achieving financial success and material wealth. In general, a person who is not financially successful or materially wealthy is not as valued in our society as someone who is (see Kasser, 2002, 2004).

Therapy as morality

Looked at in this way, it is also evident that the answer to the question of how to do therapy is not necessarily just an evidence-based one, but also a question of values and morality (see Christopher, 1996):

> When, as counselors, we interact with clients or engage in research or theorizing, we will be adopting a stance. This stance will be a moral stance, presupposing a moral vision. Whether we admit it or not in our work with clients, we are engaging in conversation about the good. Ultimately, counseling is part of a cultural discussion about ethos and world view, about the good life and the good person, and about moral visions.
>
> (Christopher, 1996, p. 24)

We are excited at the thought of the new possibilities for practice that the positive psychology approach promises to open up. We can imagine a very different healthcare system if it was based on the principles of positive psychology and the view that it is the client and not the therapist who knows best.

Recently, Totton (2004) has talked about how the profession of therapy has begun to seemingly diverge along two different paths. The first he refers to as 'expert systems' approach, which he says has evolved to cope with the demands for expertise derived through quantitative research into outcomes and effectiveness. The second he refers to as the 'local knowledge' approach, which he says has evolved to provide understanding, wisdom, and self-knowledge:

> [T]he realisation that although we all (currently) call ourselves therapists, what we are doing is in fact quite different. We can, if we choose, both accuse each other of 'not really doing psychotherapy'. Or we can recognise that, by accident of history – more specifically, by the opening up of a fault line that has always existed within the practice of therapy – two different activities have ended up bearing the same name. Maybe one or both of us will have to give up the name. But these two activities – the practice of psychological truth, and the practice of psychological helping – are both worthy, both valuable, and should both continue.
>
> (Totton, 2004, p. 8)

Our view is that these faultlines that Totton discusses have their origins in the fundamental assumptions we discussed in Chapter 2, but as we have seen earlier in this chapter, we think that the seeking of truth is helping, but helping is not seeking of truth.

Reflective practice

Inevitably, morality calls for reflection. There have been recent trends within psychology for a greater emphasis on reflective practice (see Proctor, 2005), but that reflection must be both professional and political if it is to be able to adopt a moral stance. As we have shown earlier, too often psychology can proceed without a full awareness of its inherent assumptions, values, and biases. Hence, we have tried to delineate what these may be for positive psychology as a basic science, and particularly applied positive psychology as a therapeutic practice.

The idea that there is a need for specific treatments for specific disorders currently runs to the core of how people are trained as psychologists, but we have seen that not everyone accepts this as valid (Bozarth, 1998; Bozarth & Motomasa, 2005). Mearns (1994), for example, is sceptical of the idea that working with particular client groups or issues requires prior training in that group or issue. Although there are contexts in which previous experience may be useful, for example in working with children, we would generally concur with Mearns (1994), and we would argue that training in techniques for specific problems has been overemphasised, at the expense of experiential learning toward our own authenticity and ability to accept others for who they are, and to be alongside another person and to understand the world through their eyes. As we have seen, most of the success in therapy comes through the client's own resources, and their relationship with the therapist as a facilitator of those resources (Bozarth, 1998; Bozarth & Motomasa, 2005; Hubble & Miller, 2004; Wampold, 2001). As such, it is the qualities of the therapist, their empathy and their congruence that should be the focus of training, not so much the techniques they use.

Thus, the positive therapy approach raises questions about the nature of therapist training programmes. The conclusions that we reach about the nature of therapy lead us to think that much of current professional psychology training is misguided with its emphasis on diagnosis and technique. Rather, what we would want to see is emphasis on the emotional intelligence of the therapist and their ability to develop authentic relationships. In this way, personal development should be central to training.

Conclusion

We started this book by asking about the implications of positive psychology for therapy. We have found that the current positive psychology movement raises questions about our fundamental assumptions about human nature. We propose a positive therapeutic approach based on the concept of the actualising tendency as the motivational force for optimal human development. This approach to therapy has a lineage to the humanistic psychology tradition, and to the work of Carl Rogers and Abraham Maslow in particular. The idea that the psyche contains its own natural or inherent principles that promote growth, integration, and the resolution of psychological inconsistencies and conflicts is, as we have shown, not a new one. However, it is a powerful idea that resonates with positive psychological principles and is supported by emerging theory and research.

Our approach to positive therapy might be seen as standing in contrast to some of the other recent developments in positive psychology that are more goal oriented interventions using techniques derived from cognitive-behavioural therapy. However, we do not see conflict as necessary here, because what we are offering is at a different theoretical level to these other technique-based approaches. The person-centred approach is not a collection of techniques, it is a meta-theory of personality, human functioning, and optimal development, that provides a framework for therapeutic work within which a range of therapist styles may coexist, from the more classical client-centred therapist at one end, to the more integrated process directed approaches at the other (see Sanders, 2004). What we would say is that it is not so much about what the therapist does, but rather it is about how they do it. Therapists who value and accept their clients as agents of self-determination and their own best experts are doing what we would call person-centred positive therapy.

The person-centred approach to positive therapy is an idea with revolutionary implications for therapy, suggesting as it does that the task of the therapist is to help the client to hear their own voice. We believe that therapy based on positive psychology and person-centred principles needs to be self-reflective of its fundamental assumptions, holistic and integrative of the negative and positive aspects of human experience, and aware of its social and political context. Finally, we are left with a research agenda around the nature of an innate motivational tendency toward growth and development and the social environmental conditions that are able to release this inner tendency. These are research questions of profound value, since they offer insights into the fundamentals of human nature as viewed from a positive psychological perspective.

We hope that you have enjoyed this journey with us, and that you too might share some of the passion and belief that we hold for the person-centred approach and positive therapy, and its ability to facilitate better ways of living for us all.

References

Abraido-Lanza, A. F., Guier, C., & Colon, R. M. (1998). Psychological thriving among Latinas with chronic illness. *Journal of Social Issues*, *54*, 405–424.

Ackerman, S. J., & Hilsenroth, M. J. (2003). A review of therapist characteristics and techniques positively impacting the therapeutic alliance. *Clinical Psychology Review*, *23*, 1–33.

Adler, A. (1927). *The practice and theory of individual psychology*. New York: Harcourt, Brace & World.

Affleck, G., & Tennen, H. (1996). Construing benefits from adversity: Adaptational significance and dispositional underpinnings. *Journal of Personality*, *64*, 899–922.

Affleck, G., Tennen, H., Croog, S., & Levine, S. (1987). Causal attribution, perceived benefits, and morbidity after a heart attack: An 8-year study. *Journal of Consulting and Clinical Psychology*, *55*, 29–35.

Albee, G. W. (2000). The Boulder model's fatal flaw. *American Psychologist*, *55*, 247–248.

Aldwin, C. M. (1994). Transformational coping. In C. M. Aldwin (Ed.), *Stress, coping, and development* (pp. 240–269). New York: Guilford.

American Psychiatric Association (1980). *Diagnostic and statistical manual of mental disorders (3rd edition)*. Washington, DC: American Psychiatric Press.

American Psychiatric Association (1994). *Diagnostic and statistical manual of mental disorders (4th edition)*. Washington, DC: American Psychiatric Press.

American Psychiatric Association (2000). *Diagnostic and statistical manual of mental disorders (4th edition, text revision)*. Washington, DC: American Psychiatric Press.

Andrews, F. M., & Withey, S. B. (1976). *Social indicators of well-being: America's perception of life quality*. New York: Plenum.

Angyal, A. (1941). *Foundations for a science of personality*. New York: Commonwealth Fund.

Antonovsky, A. (1987). *Unravelling the mystery of health: How people manage stress and stay well*. San Francisco: Jossey-Bass.

Armeli, S., Gunthert, K. C., & Cohen, L. H. (2001). Stressor appraisals, coping, and post-event outcomes: The dimensionality and antecedents of stress-related growth. *Journal of Social and Clinical Psychology, 20,* 366–395.

Aspinwall, L. G., & Staudinger, U. M. (Eds.) (2003). *A psychology of human strengths: Fundamental questions and future directions for a positive psychology*. Washington, DC: American Psychological Association.

Assor, A., Roth, G., & Deci, E. L. (2004). The emotional costs of parents' conditional regard: A self-determination theory analysis. *Journal of Personality, 72,* 47–88.

Baker, N. (2004). Experiential person-centred therapy. In P. Sanders (Ed.), *The tribes of the person-centred nation: An introduction to the schools of therapy related to the person-centred approach* (pp. 67–94). Ross-on-Wye: PCCS Books.

Baltes, P. B., & Staudinger, U. M. (2000). Wisdom: A metaheuristic (pragmatic) to orchestrate mind and virtue toward excellence. *American Psychologist, 55,* 122–136.

Baltes, P. B., Gluck, J., & Kunzmann, U. (2002). Wisdom: Its structure and function in regulating successful lifespan development. In C. R. Snyder, & S. J. Lopez (Eds.), *Handbook of positive psychology* (pp. 327–347). New York: Oxford University Press.

Barret-Kruse, C. (1994). Brief counseling: A user's guide for traditionally trained counsellors. *International Journal for the Advancement of Counselling, 17,* 109–115.

Barrett-Lennard, G. T. (1986). The relationship inventory now: Issues and advances in theory, method and use. In L. S. Greenberg, & W. M. Pinsof (Eds.), *The psychotherapeutic process: A research handbook* (pp. 439–476). New York: Guilford.

Barrett-Lennard, G. T. (1998). *Carl Rogers' helping system: Journey and substance*. London: Sage.

Best, M., Streisand, R., Catania, L., & Kazak, A. E. (2001). Parental distress during pediatric leukemia and posttraumatic stress symptoms (PTSS) after treatment ends. *Journal of Pediatric Psychology, 26,* 299–307.

Bohart, A. C., O'Hara, M., & Leitner, L. M. (1998). Empirically violated treatments: Disenfranchisement of humanistic and other psychotherapies. *Psychotherapy Research, 8,* 141–157.

Bolt, M. (2004). *Pursuing human strengths: A positive psychology guide*. New York: Worth.

Bozarth, J. (1998). *Person-centred therapy: A revolutionary paradigm*. Ross-on-Wye: PCCS Books.

Bozarth, J. D. (1991). Person-centered assessment. *Journal of Counseling and Development*, 69, 458–461.

Bozarth, J. D., & Brodley, B. T. (1984). Client-centered/person-centered psychotherapy: A statement of understanding. *Person-centered Review*, 1, 262–265.

Bozarth, J. D., & Motomasa, N. (2005). Searching for the core: The interface of client-centred principles with other therapies. In S. Joseph, & R. Worsley (Eds.), *Person-centred psychopathology: A positive psychology of mental health*. Ross-on-Wye: PCCS Books.

Bozarth, J. D., & Wilkins, P. (Eds.), (2001). *Rogers' therapeutic conditions: Evolution, theory and practice. Volume 3: Unconditional positive regard*. Ross-on-Wye: PCCS Books.

Brazier, D. (1993). Introduction. In D. Brazier (Ed.), *Beyond Carl Rogers: Towards a psychotherapy for the 21st century*. London: Constable.

Brazier, D. (1995). *Zen therapy*. London: Constable.

Bretherton, R., & Ørner, R. (2003). Positive psychotherapy in disguise. *The Psychologist*, 16, 136–137.

Bretherton, R., & Ørner, R. J. (2004). Positive psychology and psychotherapy: An existential approach. In P. A. Linley, & S. Joseph (Eds.), *Positive psychology in practice* (pp. 420–430). Hoboken, NJ: John Wiley & Sons.

Brickman, P., & Campbell, D. T. (1971). Hedonic relativism and planning the good society. In M. H. Appley (Ed.), *Adaptation-level theory: A symposium* (pp. 287–302). New York: Academic Press.

Brodley, B. T. (2005a). Client-centred values limit the application of research findings – an issue for discussion. In S. Joseph, & R. Worsley (Eds.), *Person-centred psychopathology: A positive psychology of mental health* (pp. 310–316). Ross-on-Wye: PCCS Books.

Brodley, B. T. (2005b). About the non-directive attitude. In B. E. Levitt (Ed.), *Embracing non-directivity: Reassessing person-centred theory and practice in the 21st century* (pp. 1–4). Ross-on-Wye: PCCS Books.

Brown, K. W., & Ryan, R. M. (2003). The benefits of being present: mindfulness and its role in psychological well-being. *Journal of Personality and Social Psychology*, 84, 822–848.

Brown, K. W., & Ryan, R. M. (2004). Fostering healthy self-regulation from within and without: A self-determination theory perspective. In P. A. Linley & S. Joseph (Eds.), *Positive psychology in practice* (pp. 105–124). Hoboken, NJ: John Wiley & Sons.

Calhoun, L. G., & Tedeschi, R. G. (1999). *Facilitating posttraumatic growth: A clinician's guide*. Mahwah, NJ: Lawrence Erlbaum.

Calhoun, L. G., Cann, A., Tedeschi, R. G., & McMillan, J. (2000). A correlational test of the relationship between posttraumatic growth, religion, and cognitive processing. *Journal of Traumatic Stress*, 13, 521–527.

Cameron, K. S., Dutton, J. E., & Quinn, R. E. (Eds.) (2003). *Positive organizational scholarship: Foundations of a new discipline.* San Francisco: Berrett-Koehler.

Carr, A. (2003). *Positive psychology: The science of happiness and human strengths.* London: Brunner-Routledge.

Carver, C. S., & Baird, E. (1998). The American dream revisited: Is it *what* you want or *why* you want it that matters? *Psychological Science, 9,* 289–292.

Chan, R., & Joseph, S. (2000). Dimensions of personality, domains of aspiration, and subjective well-being. *Personality and Individual Differences, 28,* 347–354.

Chirkov, V., Ryan, R. M., Kim, Y., & Kaplan, U. (2003). Differentiating autonomy from individualism and independence: A self-determination perspective on internalization of cultural orientations, gender, and well-being. *Journal of Personality and Social Psychology, 84,* 97–110.

Christopher, J. C. (1996). Counseling's inescapable moral visions. *Journal of Counseling and Development, 75,* 17–25.

Christopher, J. C. (1999). Situating psychological well-being: Exploring the cultural roots of its theory and research. *Journal of Counseling and Development, 77,* 141–152.

Christopher, J. C. (2003, October). *The good in positive psychology.* Paper presented at the Second International Positive Psychology Summit, Washington, DC.

Christopher, M. (2004). A broader view of trauma: A biopsychosocial-evolutionary view of the role of the traumatic stress response in the emergence of pathology and/or growth. *Clinical Psychology Review, 24,* 75–98.

Collins, R. L., Taylor, S. E., & Skokan, L. A. (1990). A better world or a shattered vision? Changes in life perspectives following victimization. *Social Cognition, 8,* 263–285.

Compton, W. C. (2004). *An introduction to positive psychology.* Belmont, CA: Wadsworth.

Compton, W. C., Smith, M. L., Cornish, K. A., & Qualls, D. L. (1996). Factor structure of mental health measures. *Journal of Personality and Social Psychology, 71,* 406–413.

Cooper, M. (2004). Existential therapies. In P. Sanders (2004). *The tribes of the person-centred nation: An introduction to the schools of therapy related to the person-centred approach* (pp. 95–124). Ross-on-Wye: PCCS Books.

Cooper, M. (2005). From self-objectification to self-affirmation: The 'I–me' and 'I–self' relation stances. In S. Joseph, & R. Worsley (Eds.), *Person-centred psychopathology: A positive psychology of mental health* (pp. 60–74). Ross-on-Wye: PCCS Books.

Corcoran, K., & Fischer, J. (2000). *Measures for clinical practice (2nd edition)*. New York: Free Press.

Cordova, M. J., Cunningham, L. L. C., Carlson, C. R., & Andrykowski, M. (2001). Posttraumatic growth following breast cancer: A controlled comparison study. *Health Psychology, 20,* 176–185.

Cornelius-White, J. H. D. (2002). The phoenix of empirically supported therapy relationships: The overlooked person-centered basis. *Psychotherapy: Theory/Research/Practice/Training, 39,* 219–222.

Creamer, M., Burgess, P., & Pattison, P. (1992). Reaction to trauma: A cognitive processing model. *Journal of Abnormal Psychology, 101,* 452–459.

Csikszentmihalyi, M. (1990). *Flow: The psychology of optimal experience*. New York: Harper & Row.

Csikszentmihalyi, M. (1997). *Finding flow: The psychology of engagement with everday life*. New York: Basic Books.

Csikszentmihalyi, M. (1999). If we are so rich, why aren't we happy? *American Psychologist, 54,* 821–827.

Csikszentmihalyi, M., & Rochberg-Halton, E. (1981). *The meaning of things. Domestic symbols and the self*. Cambridge, MA: Cambridge University Press.

Curbow, B., Legro, M. W., Baker, F., Wingard, J. R., & Somerfield, M. R. (1993). Loss and recovery themes of long-term survivors of bone marrow transplants. *Journal of Psychosocial Oncology, 10,* 1–20.

Danoff-Burg, S., & Revenson, T. A. (2005). Benefit-finding among patients with rheumatoid arthritis: Positive effects on interpersonal relationships. *Journal of Behavioral Medicine, 28,* 91–103.

Davis, C. G., Nolen-Hoeksema, S., & Larson, J. (1998). Making sense of loss and benefiting from the experience: Two construals of meaning. *Journal of Personality and Social Psychology, 75,* 561–574.

DeCarvalho, R. (1991). *The founders of humanistic psychology*. New York: Praeger.

Deci, E. L., & Ryan, R. M. (1985). *Intrinsic motivation and self-determination in human behavior*. New York: Plenum.

Deci, E. L., & Ryan, R. M. (1991). A motivational approach to self: Integration in personality. In R. Dienstbier (Ed.), *Nebraska symposium on motivation, Volume 38: Perspectives on motivation* (pp. 237–288). Lincoln, NE: University of Nebraska Press.

Deci, E. L., & Ryan, R. M. (2000). The 'what' and 'why' of goal pursuits: Human needs and the self-determination of behavior. *Psychological Inquiry, 4,* 227–268.

Deci, E. L., & Vansteenkiste, M. (2004). Self-determination theory and basic need satisfaction: Understanding human development in positive psychology. *Ricerche di psicologia: Special issue in positive psychology, 27,* 23–40.

Deci, E. L., Koestner, R., & Ryan, R. M. (1999). A meta-analytic review of experiments examining the effects of extrinsic rewards on intrinsic motivation. *Psychological Bulletin, 25,* 627–668.

Delle Fave, A., & Massimini, F. (2004). Bringing subjectivity into focus: Optimal experiences, life themes, and person-centered rehabilitation. In P. A. Linley, & S. Joseph (Eds.), *Positive psychology in practice* (pp. 581–597). Hoboken, NJ: John Wiley & Sons.

Department of Health (2000). *The NHS cancer plan.* London: Department of Health.

Deurzen, E. (1998). *Beyond psychotherapy.* Psychotherapy Section Newsletter of the British Psychological Society, 23, 4–18.

Diener, E. (2003, October). *Critiques and limitations of positive psychology.* Roundtable discussion at the Second International Positive Psychology Summit, Washington, DC.

Diener, E., & Seligman, M. E. P. (2004). Beyond money: Toward an economy of well-being. *Psychological Science in the Public Interest, 5,* 1–31.

Donlevy, J. G. (1996). Jung's contribution to adult development: The difficult and misunderstood path of individuation. *Journal of Humanistic Psychology, 36,* 92–108.

Draucker, C. (1992). Construing benefit from a negative experience of incest. *Western Journal of Nursing Research, 14,* 343–357.

Duncan, B., & Miller, S. (2000). *The heroic client: Doing client-directed, outcome informed therapy.* San Francisco: Jossey-Bass.

Edmonds, S., & Hooker, K. (1992). Perceived changes in life meaning following bereavement. *Omega, 25,* 307–318.

Eisenberg, N., & Ota Wang, V. (2003). Toward a positive psychology: Social developmental and cultural contributions. In L. G. Aspinwall, & U. M. Staudinger (Eds.), *A psychology of human strengths: Fundamental questions and future directions for a positive psychology* (pp. 117–129). Washington, DC: American Psychological Association.

Elder, G. H., Jr, & Clipp, E. C. (1989). Combat experience and emotional health: Impairment and resilience in later life. *Journal of Personality, 57,* 311–341.

Epel, E. S., McEwen, B. S., & Ickovics, J. R. (1998). Embodying psychological thriving: Physical thriving in response to stress. *Journal of Social Issues, 54,* 301–322.

Farber, B. A., Brink, D. C., & Raskin, P. M. (Eds.) (1996). *The psychotherapy of Carl Rogers: Cases and commentary.* New York: Guilford.

Fava, G. A. (1997). Conceptual obstacles to research progress in affective disorders. *Psychotherapy and Psychosomatics, 66,* 283–285.

Fava, G. A. (1999). Well-being therapy. *Psychotherapy and Psychosomatics, 68,* 171–178.

Fava, G. A. (2000). Cognitive behavioral therapy. In M. Fink (Ed.), *Encyclopedia of stress* (pp. 484–497). San Diego, CA: Academic Press.

Fava, G. A., Rafanelli, C., Cazzaro, M., Conti, S., & Grandi, S. (1998a). Well-being therapy: A novel psychotherapeutic approach for residual symptoms of affective disorders. *Psychological Medicine, 28,* 475–480.

Fava, G. A., Rafanelli, C., Grandi, S., Conti, S., & Belluardo, P. (1998b). Prevention of recurrent depression with cognitive-behavioral therapy. *Archives of General Psychiatry, 55,* 816–820.

Fava, G. A., Ruini, C., Rafanelli, C., & Grandi, S. (2002). Cognitive behavior approach to loss of clinical effect during long-term antidepressant treatment. *American Journal of Psychiatry, 159,* 2094–2095.

Fava, G. A., Ruini, C., Rafanelli, C., Finos, L., Salmaso, L., Mangelli, L., & Sirigatti, S. (2005). Well-being therapy of generalized anxiety disorder. *Psychotherapy and Psychosomatics, 74,* 26–30.

Finkel, N. J. (1975). Stress, traumas and trauma resolution. *American Journal of Community Psychology, 3,* 173–178.

Foa, E. B., & Kozak, M. J. (1986). Emotional processing of fear: Exposure to corrective information. *Psychological Bulletin, 99,* 20–35.

Foa, E. B., & Rothbaum, B. O. (1998). *Treating the trauma of rape: Cognitive-behavioral therapy for PTSD.* New York: Guilford.

Foa, E. B., Keane, T. M., & Friedman, M. J. (Eds.) (2000). *Effective treatments for PTSD: Practice guidelines from the International Society for Traumatic Stress Studies.* New York: Guilford.

Follette, W. C., Linnerooth, P. J. N., & Ruckstuhl, L. E. (2001). Positive psychology: A clinical behavior analytic perspective. *Journal of Humanistic Psychology, 41,* 102–134.

Fontana, A., & Rosenheck, R. (1998). Psychological benefits and liabilities of traumatic exposure in the war zone. *Journal of Traumatic Stress, 11,* 485–505.

Ford, J. G. (1991). Rogerian self-actualization: A clarification of meaning. *Journal of Humanistic Psychology, 31,* 101–111.

Frankel, M., & Sommerbeck, L. (2005). Two Rogers and congruence: The emergence of therapist-centred therapy and the demise of client-centred therapy. In B. E. Levitt (Ed.), *Embracing nondirectivity: Reassessing person-centred theory and practice in the 21st century* (pp. 40–61). Ross-on-Wye: PCCS Books.

Frankl, V. (1963). *Man's search for meaning: An introduction to logotherapy.* New York: Pocket Books.

Frazier, P. A., & Burnett, J. W. (1994). Immediate coping strategies among rape victims. *Journal of Counseling and Development, 72,* 633–639.

Frazier, P., Conlon, A., & Glaser, T. (2001). Positive and negative life changes following sexual assault. *Journal of Consulting and Clinical Psychology, 69,* 1048–1055.

Frazier, P., Tashiro, T., Berman, M., Steger, M., & Long, J. (2004). Correlates of levels and patterns of positive life changes following sexual assault. *Journal of Consulting and Clinical Psychology, 72*, 19–30.

Fredrickson, B. L. (1998). What good are positive emotions? *Review of General Psychology, 2*, 300–319.

Fredrickson, B. L. (2001). The role of positive emotions in positive psychology: The broaden-and-build theory of positive emotions. *American Psychologist, 56*, 218–226.

Fredrickson, B. L., & Levenson, R. W. (1998). Positive emotions speed recovery from the cardiovascular sequelae of negative emotions. *Cognition and Emotion, 12*, 191–220.

Friedli, K., King, M., Lloyd, M., & Horder, J. (1997). Randomised controlled assessment of non-directive psychotherapy versus routine general practitioner care. *Lancet, 350*, 1662–1665.

Fromm, E. (1976). *To have or to be?* New York: Harper & Row.

Fromm, K., Andrykowski, M. A., & Hunt, J. (1996). Positive and negative psychosocial sequelae of bone marrow transplantation: Implications for quality of life assessment. *Journal of Behavioral Medicine, 19*, 221–240.

Gable, S. L., & Haidt, J. (2005). What (and why) is positive psychology? *Review of General Psychology, 9*, 103–110.

Gendlin, E. T. (1996). *Focusing-oriented psychotherapy: A manual of the experiential method*. New York: Guilford.

Geuter, U. (1992). The professionalism of psychology in Nazi Germany. Cambridge: Cambridge University Press.

Goldstein, K. (1939). *The organism*. New York: American Books.

Grant, B. (2004). The imperative of ethical justification in psychotherapy: The special case of client-centered therapy. *Person-Centered and Experiential Psychotherapies, 3*, 152–165.

Greenberg, L. S., Rice, L. N., & Elliott, R. (1993). *Facilitating emotional change: the moment by moment process*. New York: Guilford.

Greening, T. (2001). Commentary. *Journal of Humanistic Psychology, 41*, 4–7.

Grossman, P., Niemann, L., Schmidt, S., & Walach, H. (2004). Mindfulness-based stress reduction and health benefits. *Journal of Psychosomatic Medicine, 57*, 35–43.

Hagan, T., & Smail, D. (1997a). Power mapping – I. Background and basic methodology. *Journal of Community and Applied Social Psychology, 7*, 257–267.

Hagan, T., & Smail, D. (1997b). Power mapping – II. Practical application: The example of sexual abuse. *Journal of Community and Applied Social Psychology, 7*, 269–284.

Hansard, C. (2001). *The Tibetan art of living: Wise body, wise mind, wise life*. London: Hodder & Stoughton.

Harlow, H. F. (1953). Mice, monkeys, men, and motives. *Psychological Review, 60*, 23–32.

Harter, S., Marold, D. B., Whitesell, N. R., & Cobbs, G. (1996). A model of the effects of parent and peer support on adolescent false self behavior. *Child Development, 67*, 360–374.

Harvey, J. H. (2001). The psychology of loss as a lens to positive psychology. *American Behavioral Scientist, 44*, 838–853.

Haugh, S., & Merry, T. (Eds.) (2001). *Rogers' therapeutic conditions: Evolution, theory and practice. Volume 2: Empathy*. Ross-on-Wye: PCCS Books.

Heelas, P., & Lock, A. (Eds.) (1981). *Indigenous psychologies: The anthropology of the self*. New York: Academic.

Hegel, G. W. F. (1931). *The phenomenology of mind*. (Trans. J. B. Baillie, 2nd ed.). (Original work published 1807.) London: Allen & Unwin.

Held, B. S. (2002). The tyranny of the positive attitude in America: Observation and speculation. *Journal of Clinical Psychology, 58*, 965–992.

Held, B. S. (2003, October). *Critiques and limitations of positive psychology*. Roundtable discussion at the Second International Positive Psychology Summit, Washington, DC.

Herman, J. L. (1992). *Trauma and recovery: From domestic abuse to political terror*. London: Pandora.

Hodges, T. D., & Clifton, D. O. (2004). Strengths based development in practice. In P. A. Linley, & S. Joseph (Eds.), *Positive psychology in practice* (pp. 256–268). Hoboken, NJ: John Wiley & Sons.

Horney, K. (1951). *Neurosis and human growth: The struggle toward self-realization*. London: Routledge & Kegan Paul.

Horowitz, M. J. (1982). Psychological processes induced by illness, injury, and loss. In T. Millon., C. Green., & R. Meagher (Eds.), *Handbook of clinical health psychology* (pp. 53–68). New York: Plenum.

Horowitz, M. J. (1986). *Stress response syndromes*. Northville, NJ: Jason Aronson.

Hubble, M. A., & Miller, S. D. (2004). The client: Psychotherapy's missing link for promoting a positive psychology. In P. A. Linley, & S. Joseph (Eds.), *Positive psychology in practice* (pp. 335–353). Hoboken, NJ: John Wiley & Sons.

Huppert, F. A. (2004). A population approach to positive psychology: The potential for population interventions to promote well-being and prevent disorder. In P. A. Linley, & S. Joseph (Eds.), *Positive psychology in practice* (pp. 693–709). Hoboken, NJ: John Wiley & Sons.

Jaffe, D. T. (1985). Self-renewal: Personal transformation following extreme trauma. *Journal of Humanistc Psychology, 25*, 99–124.

James, W. (1902). *The varieties of religious experience: A study in human nature*. New York: Longman, Green.

Janoff-Bulman, R. (1989). Assumptive worlds and the stress of traumatic events: Applications of the schema construct. *Social Cognition, 7,* 113–136.

Janoff-Bulman, R. (1992). *Shattered assumptions: Towards a new psychology of trauma*. New York: Free Press.

Janoff-Bulman, R., & McPherson Frantz, C. (1997). *The impact of trauma on meaning: From meaningless world to meaningful life*. In M. Power, & C. R. Brewin (Eds.), *The transformation of meaning in psychological therapies*. Chichester: John Wiley & Sons.

Joseph, S. (1999). Attributional processes, coping, and post-traumatic stress disorders. In W. Yule (Ed.), *Post-traumatic stress disorders: Concepts and therapy* (pp. 51–70). Chichester: John Wiley & Sons.

Joseph, S. (2001). *Psychopathology and therapeutic approaches: An introduction*. Houndmills: Palgrave Macmillan.

Joseph, S. (2003a). Client-centred psychotherapy: Why the client knows best. *The Psychologist, 16,* 304–307.

Joseph, S. (2003b). Person-centred approach to understanding posttraumatic stress. *Person-centred Practice, 11,* 70–75.

Joseph, S. (2004). Client-centred therapy, posttraumatic stress, and posttraumatic growth: Theoretical perspectives and practical implications. *Psychology and Psychotherapy: Theory, Research and Practice, 77,* 101–120.

Joseph, S. (2005). Understanding posttraumatic stress from the person-centred perspective. In S. Joseph, and R. Worsley (Eds.), *Person-centred psychopathology: A positive psychology of mental health* (pp. 190–201). Ross-on-Wye: PCCS Books.

Joseph, S., & Lewis, C. A. (1998). The depression–happiness scale: Reliability and validity of a bipolar self-report scale. *Journal of Clinical Psychology, 54,* 537–544.

Joseph, S., & Linley, P. A. (2004). Positive therapy: A positive psychological theory of therapeutic practice. In P. A. Linley, & S. Joseph (Eds.), *Positive psychology in practice* (pp. 354–368). Hoboken, NJ: John Wiley & Sons.

Joseph, S., & Linley, P. A. (2005a). Positive psychological approaches to therapy. *Counselling and Psychotherapy Research, 5,* 5–10.

Joseph, S., & Linley, P. A. (2005b). Positive adjustment to threatening events: An organismic valuing theory of growth through adversity. *Review of General Psychology, 9,* 262–280.

Joseph, S., & Worsley, R. (Eds.) (2005a). *Person-centred psychopathology: A positive psychology of mental health*. Ross-on-Wye: PCCS Books.

Joseph, S., & Worsley, R. (2005b). A positive psychology of mental health: The person centred perspective. In S. Joseph, & R. Worsley (Eds.), *Person-centred psychopathology: A positive psychology of mental health* (pp. 348–357). Ross-on-Wye: PCCS Books.

Joseph, S., Williams, R., & Yule, W. (1993). Changes in outlook following disaster: The preliminary development of a measure to assess positive and negative responses. *Journal of Traumatic Stress, 6,* 271–279.

Joseph, S., Williams, R., & Yule, W. (1995). Psychosocial perspective on Posttraumatic stress. *Clinical Psychology Review, 15,* 515–544.

Joseph, S., Williams, R., & Yule, W. (1997). *Understanding posttraumatic stress: A psychosocial perspective on PTSD and treatment.* Chichester: John Wiley & Sons.

Joseph, S., Linley, P. A., Harwood, J., Lewis, C. A., & McCollam, P. (2004). Rapid assessment of well-being: The short depression–happiness scale. *Psychology and Psychotherapy: Theory, Research, and Practice, 77,* 1–14.

Joseph, S., Linley, P. A., Andrews, L., Harris, G., Howle, B., Woodward, C., & Shevlin, M. (2005). Assessing positive and negative changes in the aftermath of adversity: Psychometric evaluation of the changes in outlook questionnaire. *Psychological Assessment, 17,* 70–80.

Joseph, S., Linley, P. A., Shevlin, M., Goodfellow, B., & Butler, L. (2006). Assessing positive and negative changes in the aftermath of adversity: A short form of the changes in outlook questionnaire. *Journal of Loss and Trauma 11,* 85–99.

Judge, T. A., Thoresen, C. J., Bono, J. E., & Patton, G. K. (2001). The job satisfaction-job performance relationship: A qualitative and quantitative review. *Psychological Bulletin, 127,* 376–407.

Jung, C. G. (1933). *Modern man in search of a soul.* New York: Harcourt, Brace, & World.

Kahneman, D. (1999). Objective happiness. In D. Kahneman, E. Diener, & N. Schwarz (Eds.), *Well-being: The foundations of hedonic psychology* (pp. 3–25). New York: Russell Sage Foundation.

Kasser, T. (2002). *The high price of materialism.* Cambridge, MA: MIT Press.

Kasser, T. (2004). The good life or the goods life? Positive psychology and personal well-being in the culture of consumption. In P. A. Linley, & S. Joseph (Eds.), *Positive psychology in practice* (pp. 55–67). Hoboken, NJ: John Wiley & Sons.

Kasser, T., & Ryan, R. M. (1993). A dark side of the American dream: Correlates of financial success as a central life aspiration. *Journal of Personality and Social Psychology, 65,* 410–422.

Kasser, T., & Ryan, R. M. (1996). Further examining the American dream: Differential correlates of intrinsic and extrinsic goals. *Personality and Social Psychology Bulletin, 22,* 280–287.

Kasser, T., Ryan, R. M., Zax, M., & Sameroff, A. J. (1995). The relations of material and social environments to adolescents' materialistic and prosocial values. *Developmental Psychology, 31*, 907–914.

Kauffman, C. (2005). *You are just p.e.r.f.e.c.t. A positive psychology perspective of multiple resources.* Paper presented at the American Psychological Association, Washington, DC.

Kauffman, C., & Scoular, A. (2004). Toward a positive psychology of exectutive coaching. In P. A. Linley & S. Joseph (Eds.), *Positive psychology in practice* (pp. 287–302). Hoboken, NJ: John Wiley & Sons.

Kearney, A. (1996). *Counselling, class and politics: Undeclared influences in therapy.* Ross-on-Wye: PCCS Books.

Kekes, J. (1995). *Moral wisdom and good lives.* Ithaca, NY: Cornell University Press.

Kessler, B. G. (1987). Bereavement and personal growth. *Journal of Humanistic Psychology, 27*, 228–247.

Keyes, C. L. M., & Haidt, J. (Eds.) (2002). *Flourishing: Positive psychology and the life well-lived.* Washington, DC: American Psychological Association.

Keyes, C. L. M., Shmotkin, D., & Ryff, C. D. (2002). Optimizing well-being: The empirical encounter of two traditions. *Journal of Personality and Social Psychology, 82*, 1007–1022.

Kidner, D. (2001). Silence is a political act: Letters to the editor. *The Psychologist, 14*, 178.

King, M., Sibbald, B., Ward, E., Bower, P., Lloyd, M., Gabbay, M., & Byford, S. (2000). Randomised controlled trail of non-directive counselling, cognitive behaviour therapy, and usual general practitioner care in the management of depression as well as mixed anxiety and depression in primary care. *British Medical Journal, 321*, 1383–1388.

Kirschenbaum, H. (2004). Carl Rogers's life and work: An assessment on the 100th anniversary of his birth. *Journal of Counseling and Development, 82*, 116–124.

Kirschenbaum, H., & Henderson, V. C. (Eds.) (1989). *The Carl Rogers reader.* Boston, MA: Houghton-Mifflin.

Koenig, H. G., Pargament, K. I., & Nielsen, J. (1998). Religious coping and health status in medically ill hospitalized older adults. *Journal of Nervous and Mental Disease, 186*, 513–521.

Korchin, S. J. (1976). *Modern clinical psychology.* New York: Basic Books.

Krupnick, L. J., Sotsky, S. M., Simmens, S., Moyer, J., Elkin, I., Watkins, J., & Pilkonis, P. A. (1996). The role of the therapeutic alliance in psychotherapy and pharmacotherapy outcome: Findings in the National Institute of Mental Health Treatment of Depression Collaborative Research Programme. *Journal of Consulting and Clinical Psychology, 64*, 532–539.

Laerum, E., Johnsen, N., Smith, P., & Larsen, S. (1987). Can myocardial infarction induce positive changes in family relationships? *Family Practice*, 4, 302–305.

La Guardia, J. G., Ryan, R. M., Couchman, C. E., & Deci, E. L. (2000). Within-person variation in security of attachment: A self-determination theory perspective on attachment, need fulfilment, and well-being. *Journal of Personality and Social Psychology*, 79, 367–384.

Lambert, M. J. (1992). Implications of outcome research for psychotherapy integration. In J. C. Norcross, & M. R. Goldfried (Eds.), *Handbook of psychotherapy integration* (pp. 94–129). New York: Basic Books.

Larsen, J. T., Hemenover, S. H., Norris, C. J., & Cacioppo, J. T. (2003). Turning adversity to advantage: On the virtues of the coactivation of positive and negative emotions. In L. G. Aspinwall, & U. M. Staudinger (Eds.), *A psychology of human strengths: Fundamental questions and future directions for a positive psychology* (pp. 211–225). Washington, DC: American Psychological Association.

Lavender, T. (2003). Redressing the balance: The place, history and future of reflective practice in training. *Clinical Psychology*, 27, 11–15.

Lazarus, R. S. (2003). Does the positive psychology movement have legs? *Psychological Inquiry*, 14, 93–109.

Lazarus, R. S., & Folkman, S. (1984). *Stress, appraisal, and coping*. New York: Springer.

Lehman, D. R., Davis, C. G., DeLongis, A., Wortman, C. B., Bluck, S., Mandel, D. R., & Ellard, J. H. (1993). Positive and negative life changes following bereavement and their relations to adjustment. *Journal of Social and Clinical Psychology*, 12, 90–112.

Levitt, B. E. (2005a). Non-directivity: The foundational attitude. In B. E. Levitt (Ed.), *Embracing non-directivity: Reassessing person-centred theory and practice in the 21st century* (pp. 5–16). Ross-on-Wye: PCCS Books.

Levitt, B. E. (2005b). *Embracing non-directivity: Reassessing person-centred theory and practice in the 21st century*. Ross-on-Wye: PCCS Books.

Linley, P. A. (2000). Transforming psychology: The example of trauma. *The Psychologist*, 13, 353–355.

Linley, P. A. (2003). Positive adaptation to trauma: Wisdom as both process and outcome. *Journal of Traumatic Stress*, 16, 601–610.

Linley, P. A., & Harrington, S. (2006). Playing to your strengths. *The Psychologist* 19, 86–89.

Linley, P. A., & Joseph, S. (2002a). Posttraumatic growth. *Counselling and Psychotherapy Journal*, 13, 14–17.

Linley, P. A., & Joseph, S. (2002b, June). *Posttraumatic growth: The positive psychology of trauma*. Paper presented at the First European Positive Psychology Conference, Winchester, UK.

Linley, P. A., & Joseph, S. (2002c, October). *Posttraumatic growth: The apotheosis of positive psychology*. Poster presented at the First International Positive Psychology Summit, Washington, DC.

Linley, P. A., & Joseph, S. (2003). Putting it into practice. *The Psychologist, 16*, 143.

Linley, P. A., & Joseph, S. (Eds.) (2004a). *Positive psychology in practice*. Hoboken, NJ: John Wiley & Sons.

Linley, P. A., & Joseph, S. (2004b). Applied positive psychology: A new perspective for professional practice. In P. A. Linley, & S. Joseph (Eds.), *Positive psychology in practice* (pp. 3–12). Hoboken, NJ: John Wiley & Sons.

Linley, P. A., & Joseph, S. (2004c). Toward a theoretical foundation for positive psychology in practice. In P. A. Linley, & S. Joseph (Eds.), *Positive psychology in practice* (pp. 713–731). Hoboken, NJ: John Wiley & Sons.

Linley, P. A., & Joseph, S. (2004d). Positive change following trauma and adversity: A review. *Journal of Traumatic Stress, 17*, 11–21.

Linley, P. A., & Joseph, S. (2005). The human capacity for growth through adversity. *American Psychologist, 60*, 262–263.

Linley, P. A., Joseph, S., Cooper, R., Harris, S., & Meyer, C. (2003). Positive and negative changes following vicarious exposure to the September 11 terrorist attacks. *Journal of Traumatic Stress, 16*, 481–485.

Linley, P. A., Joseph, S., Harrington, S., & Wood, A. M. (2006). Positive psychology: Past, present, and (possible) future. *The Journal of Positive Psychology 1*, 3–16.

Linley, P. A., Joseph, S., & Loumidis, K. (2005). Trauma work, sense of coherence, and positive and negative changes in therapists. *Psychotherapy and Psychosomatics, 74*, 185–188.

Littlewood, R., & Lipsedge, M. (1993). *Aliens and alienists: Ethnic minorities and psychiatry (3rd edition)*. London: Routledge.

Lopez, S. J., & Snyder, C. R. (Eds.) (2003). *Positive psychological assessment: A handbook of models and measures*. Washington, DC: American Psychological Association.

Lopez, S. J., Prosser, E. C., Edwards, L. M., Magyar-Moe, J. L., Neufeld, J. E., & Rasmussen, H. N. (2002). Putting positive psychology in a multicultural context. In C. R. Snyder, & S. J. Lopez (Eds.), *Handbook of positive psychology* (pp. 700–714). New York: Oxford University Press.

Lyons, J. A. (1991). Strategies for assessing the potential for positive adjustment following trauma. *Journal of Traumatic Stress, 4*, 93–111.

Ma, S. H., & Teasdale, J. D. (2004). Mindfulness-based cognitive therapy for depression: Replication and exploration of differential relapse prevention effects. *Journal of Consulting and Clinical Psychology, 72*, 31–40.

Maddux, J. E. (2002). Stopping the 'madness': Positive psychology and the deconstruction of the illness ideology and the *DSM*. In C. R. Snyder, & S. J. Lopez (Eds.), *Handbook of positive psychology* (pp. 13–25). New York: Oxford University Press.

Maddux, J. E., Gosselin, J. T., & Winstead, B. A. (2004a). Conceptions of psychopathology: A social constructionist perspective. In J. E. Maddux, & B. A. Winstead (Eds), *Psychopathology: Foundations for a contemporary understanding*. Mahwah, NJ: Lawrence Erlbaum.

Maddux, J. E., Snyder, C. R., & Lopez, S. J. (2004b). Toward a positive clinical psychology: Deconstructing the illness ideology and constructing an ideology of human strengths and potential. In P. A. Linley, & S. Joseph (Eds.), *Positive psychology in practice* (pp. 320–334). Hoboken, NJ: John Wiley & Sons.

Marcus, G. E., & Fischer, M. M. J. (1986). *Anthropology as cultural critique: An experimental moment in the human sciences*. Chicago, IL: University of Chicago Press.

Martin, J. (2004). *Adversarial growth following cancer*. Doctor of clinical psychology thesis, University of Warwick.

Martin, D. J., Garske, J. P., & Davis, M. K. (2000). Relation of the therapeutic alliance with outcome and other variables: A meta-analytic review. *Journal of Consulting and Clinical Psychology, 68*, 438–450.

Martin, J., Tolosa, I., & Joseph, S. (2004). Adversarial growth following cancer and support from health professionals. *Health Psychology Update, 13*, 11–17.

Marzillier, J. (2004). Psychotherapy – is evidence the answer? Letters page. *The Psychologist, 17*, 625–626.

Maslow, A. H. (1954). *Motivation and personality*. New York: Harper & Row.

Maslow, A. H. (1968). *Toward a psychology of being*. New York: Van Nostrand.

Maslow, A. H. (1970). *Motivation and personality (2nd edition)*. New York: Harper & Row.

Maslow, A. H. (1993). *The farther reaches of human nature*. New York: Penguin Arkana.

May, R. (1994). Contributions of existential psychotherapy. In R. May, E. Angel, & H. F. Ellenberger (Eds.), *Existence* (pp. 37–91). Northvale, NJ: Jason Aronson. (Original work published 1958.)

McGregor, I., & Little, B. R. (1998). Personal projects, happiness, and meaning: On doing well and being yourself. *Journal of Personality and Social Psychology, 74*, 494–512.

McMillen, J. C. (1999). Better for it: How people benefit from adversity. *Social Work, 44,* 455–468.

McMillen, J. C., & Fisher, R. H. (1998). The perceived benefit scales: Measuring perceived positive life changes after negative events. *Social Work Research, 22,* 173–187.

McMillen, C., Zuravin, S., & Rideout, G. (1995). Perceived benefits from child sexual abuse. *Journal of Consulting and Clinical Psychology, 63,* 1037–1043.

McMillen, C., Howard, M. O., Nower, L., & Chung, S. (2001). Positive by-products of the struggle with chemical dependency. *Journal of Substance Abuse Treatment, 20,* 69–79.

Mearns, D. (1994). *Developing person-centred counselling.* London: Sage.

Mearns, D., & Thorne, B. (1999). *Person-centred counselling in action (2nd edition).* London: Sage.

Mearns, D., & Thorne, B. (2000). *Person-centred therapy today: New frontiers in theory and practice.* London: Sage.

Mendola, R., Tennen, H., Affleck, G., McCann, L., & Fitzgerald, T. (1990). Appraisal and adaptation among women with impaired fertility. *Cognitive Therapy and Research, 14,* 79–93.

Merry, T. (1999). *Learning and being in person-centred counselling: A textbook for discovering theory and developing practice.* Ross-on-Wye: PCCS Books.

Merry, T. (2004). Classical client-centred therapy. In P. Sanders (2004), *The tribes of the person-centred nation: An introduction to the schools of therapy related to the person-centred approach* (pp. 21–44). Ross-on-Wye: PCCS Books.

Milam, J. E., Ritt-Olson, A., & Unger, J. (in press). Posttraumatic growth among adolescents. *Journal of Adolescent Research.*

Miles, M. S., Demi, A. S., & Mostyn-Aker, P. (1984). Rescue workers' reactions following the Hyatt Hotel disaster. *Death Education, 8,* 315–331.

Miller, W. R., & C'deBaca, J. (1994). Quantum change: Toward a psychology of transformation. In T. F. Heatherton, & J. L. Weinberger (Eds.), *Can personality change?* (pp. 253–281). Washington, DC: American Psychological Association.

Milne, D. (1999). Editorial: Important differences between the 'scientist-practitioner' and the 'evidence-based practitioner'. *Clinical Psychology Forum, 133,* 5–9.

Myers, D. G. (2000). The funds, friends, and faith of happy people. *American Psychologist, 55,* 56–67.

Myers, D. G. (2004). Human connections and the good life: Balancing individuality and community in public policy. In P. A. Linley, & S. Joseph (Eds.), *Positive psychology in practice* (pp. 641–657). Hoboken, NJ: John Wiley & Sons.

Nelson-Jones, R. (1984). *Personal responsibility counselling and therapy: An integrative approach*. London: Harper & Row.

Norcross, J. C. (Ed.) (2001). Empirically supported therapy relationships: Summary of the Division 29 Task Force [Special Issue]. *Psychotherapy, 38* (4).

Norem, J. K. (2003, October). *Critiques and limitations of positive psychology*. Roundtable discussion at the Second International Positive Psychology Summit, Washington, DC.

O'Connell, B. (2001). *Solution focused stress counselling*. London: Continuum.

O'Connell, B. (2005). *Solution-focused therapy (2nd edition)*. London: Sage.

O'Connor, A. P., Wicker, C. A., & Germino, B. B. (1990). Understanding the cancer patient's search for meaning. *Cancer Nursing, 13,* 167–175.

O'Hara, M. (1997). Emancipatory therapeutic practice in a turbulent transmodern era: A work of retrieval. *Journal of Humanistic Psychology, 37,* 7–33.

O'Leary, V. E., & Ickovics, J. R. (1995). Resilience and thriving in response to challenge: An opportunity for a paradigm shift in women's health. *Women's Health: Research on Gender, Behavior, and Policy, 1,* 121–142.

Parappully, J., Rosenbaum, R., van den Daele, L., & Nzewi, E. (2002). Thriving after trauma: The experience of parents of murdered children. *Journal of Humanistic Psychology, 42,* 33–70.

Pargament, K. I., & Mahoney, A. (2002). Spirituality: Discovering and conserving the sacred. In C. R. Snyder, & S. J. Lopez (Eds.), *Handbook of positive psychology* (pp. 646–659). New York: Oxford University Press.

Pargament, K. I., Smith, B. W., Koenig, H. G., & Perez, L. (1998). Patterns of positive and negative religious coping with major life stressors. *Journal for the Scientific Study of Religion, 37,* 710–724.

Park, C. L. (1998). Stress-related growth and thriving through coping: The roles of personality and cognitive processes. *Journal of Social Issues, 54,* 267–277.

Park, C. L., Cohen, L. H., & Murch, R. (1996). Assessment and prediction of stress-related growth. *Journal of Personality, 64,* 71–105.

Parks, A. C. (2004, September–October). *Treating depressive symptoms with a positive intervention*. Poster presented at 2004 International Positive Psychology Summit.

Patterson, T., & Joseph, S. (in press). Person-centered personality theory: Support from self-determination theory and positive psychology. *Journal of Humanistic Psychology.*

Pavot, W., & Diener, E. (2004). Findings on subjective well-being: Applications to public policy, clinical interventions, and education. In P. A.

Linley, & S. Joseph (Eds.), *Positive psychology in practice* (pp. 679–692). Hoboken, NJ: John Wiley & Sons.

Peseschkian, N., & Tritt, K. (1998). Positive psychotherapy: Effectiveness study and quality assurance. *European Journal of Psychotherapy, Counselling, and Health, 1,* 93–104.

Peterson, C., & Seligman, M. E. P. (2003). Values in action (VIA) classification of strengths. Draft (January 4, 2003), retrieved from World Wide Web (www.positivepsychology.org/strengths), 15 January 2003.

Peterson, C., & Seligman, M. E. P. (2004). *Character strengths and virtues: A handbook and classification.* Washington, DC: American Psychological Association.

Prilleltensky, I. (1994). *The morals and politics of psychology: Psychological discourse and the status quo.* Albany, NY: State University of New York Press.

Proctor, G. (2005). Clinical psychology and the person-centred approach: An uncomfortable fit. In S. Joseph, & R. Worsley (Eds.), *Person-centred psychopathology: A positive psychology of mental health* (pp. 276–292). Ross-on-Wye: PCCS Books.

Prouty, G. (1990). Pre-therapy: A theoretical evolution in the person-centred/experiential psychotherapy of schizophrenia and retardation. In G. Lietaer, J. Rombauts, & R. Van Balen (Eds.), *Client-centred and experiential psychotherapy in the nineties* (pp. 645–658). Leuven: University of Leuven Press.

Prouty, G., Van Werde, D., & Portner, M. (2002). *Pre-therapy: Reaching contact-impaired clients.* Ross-on-Wye: PCCS books.

Rachman, S. (1980). Emotional processing. *Behaviour Research and Therapy, 18,* 51–60.

Rank, O. (1936). *Truth and reality: A life history of the human will.* New York: Knopf.

Raphael, B. (1986). *When disaster strikes.* Hutchinson: London.

Rathunde, K. (2001). Toward a psychology of optimal human functioning: What positive psychology can learn from the 'experiential turns' of James, Dewey, and Maslow. *Journal of Humanistic Psychology, 41,* 135–153.

Reeve, J., Nix, G., & Hamm, D. (2003). Testing models of the experience of self-determination in intrinsic motivation and the conundrum of choice. *Journal of Educational Psychology, 95,* 375–392.

Reisman, J. M. (1991). *A history of clinical psychology.* New York: Hemisphere.

Rennie, D. L. (1996). Fifteen years of doing qualitative psychotherapy process research. *British Journal of Guidance and Counselling, 24,* 317–327.

Rennie, D. L. (1998). *Person-centred counselling: An experiential approach*. London: Sage.

Resnick, S., Warmoth, A., & Serlin, I. A. (2001). The humanistic psychology and positive psychology connection: Implications for psychotherapy. *Journal of Humanistic Psychology, 41*, 73–101.

Rogers, C. R. (1942). *Counseling and psychotherapy: Newer concepts in practice*. Boston, MA: Houghton-Mifflin.

Rogers, C. R. (1951). *Client-centered therapy: Its current practice, implications and theory*. Boston, MA: Houghton-Mifflin.

Rogers, C. R. (1957). The necessary and sufficient conditions of therapeutic personality change. *Journal of Consulting Psychology, 21*, 95–103.

Rogers, C. R. (1959). A theory of therapy, personality and interpersonal relationships, as developed in the client-centered framework. In S. Koch (Ed.), *Psychology: A study of a science, Vol. 3: Formulations of the person and the social context* (pp. 184–256). New York: McGraw-Hill.

Rogers, C. R. (1961). *On becoming a person*. Boston, MA: Houghton-Mifflin.

Rogers, C. R. (1963a). The actualizing tendency in relation to 'motives' and to consciousness. In M. Jones (ed.), *Nebraska symposium on motivation, Volume 11* (pp. 1–24). Lincoln: University of Nebraska Press.

Rogers, C. R. (1963b). The concept of the fully functioning person. *Psychotherapy: Theory, Research, and Practice, 1*, 17–26.

Rogers, C. R. (1964). Toward a modern approach to values: The valuing process in the mature person. *Journal of Abnormal and Social Psychology, 68*, 160–167.

Rogers, C. R. (1969). *Freedom to learn*. Columbus, OH: Merrill.

Rogers, C. R. (1978). *Carl Rogers on personal power: Inner strength and its revolutionary impact*. London: Constable.

Rollnick, S., & Miller, W. R. (1995). What is motivational interviewing? *Behavioural and Cognitive Psychotherapy, 23*, 325–334.

Rosenhan, D. L. (1973). On being sane in insane places. *Science, 179*, 250–258.

Rosenhan, D. L. (1975). The contextual nature of psychiatric diagnosis. *Journal of Abnormal Psychology, 84*, 442–452.

Roth, S., Lebowitz, L., & DeRosa, R. R. (1997). Thematic assessment of posttraumatic stress reactions. In J. P. Wilson, & T. M. Keane (Eds.), *Assessing psychological trauma and PTSD* (pp. 512–528). New York: Guilford.

Ruini, C., & Fava, G. A. (2004). Clinical applications of well-being therapy. In P. A. Linley, & S. Joseph (Eds.), *Positive psychology in practice* (pp. 371–387). Hoboken, NJ: John Wiley & Sons.

Ryan, R. M. (1995). Psychological needs and the facilitation of integrative processes. *Journal of Personality*, *63*, 397–427.

Ryan, R. M., & Deci, E. L. (2000). Self-determination theory and the facilitation of intrinsic motivation, social development, and well-being. *American Psychologist*, *55*, 68–78.

Ryan, R. M., & Deci, E. L. (2001). On happiness and human potentials: A review of research on hedonic and eudaemonic well-being. *Annual Review of Psychology*, *52*, 141–166.

Ryff, C. D. (1989). Happiness is everything, or is it? Explorations on the meaning of psychological well-being. *Journal of Personality and Social Psychology*, *57*, 1069–1081.

Ryff, C. D., & Singer, B. H. (1996). Psychological well-being: Meaning, measurement, and implications for psychotherapy research. *Psychotherapy and Psychosomatics*, *65*, 14–23.

Ryff, C. D., & Singer, B. (2003). Ironies of the human condition: Well-being and health on the way to mortality. In L. G. Aspinwall, & U. M. Staudinger (Eds.), *A psychology of human strengths: Fundamental questions and future directions for a positive psychology* (pp. 271–287). Washington, DC: American Psychological Association.

Salovey, P., Mayer, J. D., & Caruso, D. (2002). The positive psychology of emotional intelligence. In C. R. Snyder, & S. J. Lopez (Eds.), *Handbook of positive psychology* (pp. 159–171). New York: Oxford University Press.

Salovey, P., Caruso, D., & Mayer, J. D. (2004). Emotional intelligence in practice. In P. A. Linley, & S. Joseph (Eds.), *Positive psychology in practice* (pp. 447–463). Hoboken, NJ: John Wiley & Sons.

Sanders, P. (2004). *The tribes of the person-centred nation: An introduction to the schools of therapy related to the person-centred approach.* Ross-on-Wye: PCCS Books.

Sanders, P. (2005). Principled and strategic opposition to the medicalisation of distress and all of its apparatus. In S. Joseph, & R. Worsley (Eds.), *Person-centred psychopathology: A positive psychology of mental health* (pp. 21–42). Ross-on-Wye: PCCS Books.

Schmid, P. (2005). Facilitative responsiveness: Non-directiveness from anthropological, epistemological and ethical perspectives. In B. E. Levitt (Ed.), *Embracing nondirectivity: Reassessing person-centred theory and practice in the 21st century* (pp. 75–95). Ross-on-Wye: PCCS Books.

Schwartzberg, S. S. (1993). *Struggling for meaning: How HIV-positive gay men make sense of AIDS. Professional Psychology: Research and Practice*, *24*, 483–490.

Sears, S. R., Stanton, A. L., & Danoff-Burg, S. (2003). The yellow brick road and the emerald city: Benefit finding, positive reappraisal coping, and posttraumatic growth in women with early-stage breast cancer. *Health Psychology, 22*, 487–497.

Seligman, M. E. P. (1994). *What you can change and what you can't.* New York: Knopf.

Seligman, M. E. P. (1999). The president's address. *American Psychologist, 54*, 559–562.

Seligman, M. E. P. (2001, October). *Welcome to positive psychology.* Address to the Positive Psychology Summit, Washington, DC.

Seligman, M. E. P. (2002). Positive psychology, positive prevention, and positive therapy. In C. R. Snyder, & S. J. Lopez (Eds.), *Handbook of positive psychology* (pp. 3–9). New York: Oxford University Press.

Seligman, M. E. P. (2003a). Positive psychology: Fundamental assumptions. *The Psychologist, 16*, 126–127.

Seligman, M. E. P. (2003b). *Authentic happiness: Using the new positive psychology to realize your potential for lasting fulfilment.* New York: Free Press.

Seligman, M. E. P., & Csikszentmihalyi, M. (2000). Positive psychology: An introduction. *American Psychologist, 55*, 5–14.

Seligman, M. E. P., & Peterson, C. (2003). Positive clinical psychology. In L. G. Aspinwall, & U. M. Staudinger (Eds.), *A psychology of human strengths: Fundamental questions and future directions for a positive psychology* (pp. 305–317). Washington, DC: American Psychological Association.

Seligman, M. E. P., Steen, T. A., Park, N., & Peterson, C. (2005). Positive psychology progress: Empirical validation of interventions. *American Psychologist, 60*, 410–421.

Shaw, A., Joseph, S., & Linley, P. A. (2005). Religion, spirituality and posttraumatic growth: A review. *Mental Health, Religion, and Culture, 8*, 1–11.

Sheldon, K. M., & Elliot, A. J. (1999). Goal striving, need satisfaction, and longitudinal well-being: The self-concordance model. *Journal of Personality and Social Psychology, 76*, 482–497.

Sheldon, K. M., & Houser-Marko, L. (2001). Self-concordance, goal attainment, and the pursuit of happiness: Can there be an upward spiral? *Journal of Personality and Social Psychology, 80*, 152–165.

Sheldon, K. M., & Kasser, T. (2001). Goals, congruence, and positive well-being: New empirical support for humanistic theories. *Journal of Humanistic Psychology, 41*, 30–50.

Sheldon, K. M., & King, L. (2001). Why positive psychology is necessary. *American Psychologist, 56*, 216–217.

Sheldon, K. M., & Luyubomirsky, S. (2004). Achieving sustainable new happiness: Prospects, practices, and prescriptions. In P. A. Linley, & S. Joseph (Eds.), *Positive psychology in practice* (pp. 127–145). Hoboken, NJ: John Wiley & Sons.

Sheldon, K. M., & McGregor, H. A. (2000). Extrinsic value orientation and 'the tragedy of the commons'. *Journal of Personality, 68,* 383–411.

Sheldon, K. M., Arndt, J., & Houser-Marko, L. (2003a). In search of the organismic valueing process: The human tendency to move towards beneficial goal choices. *Journal of Personality, 71,* 835–886.

Sheldon, K. M., Joiner, T. E., Pettit, J. W., & Williams, G. (2003b). Reconciling humanistic ideas and scientific clinical practice. *Clinical Psychology: Science and Practice, 10,* 302–315.

Shlien, J. M. (2003a). A criterion of psychological health. In P. Sanders (Ed.), *To lead an honourable life: Invitations to think about client-centred therapy and the person-centred approach* (pp. 15–18). Ross-on-Wye: PCCS Books.

Shlien, J. M. (2003b). Creativity and psychological health. In P. Sanders (Ed.), *To lead an honourable life: Invitations to think about client-centred therapy and the person-centred approach* (pp. 19–29). Ross-on-Wye: PCCS Books.

Shweder, R. A., & Bourne, E. J. (1984). Does the concept of the person vary cross-culturally? In R. A. Shweder, & R. A. LeVine (Eds.), *Culture theory: Essays on mind, self, and emotion* (pp. 158–199). New York: Cambridge University Press.

Siegel, K., & Schrimshaw, E. W. (2000). Perceiving benefits in adversity: Stress-related growth in women living with HIV/AIDS. *Social Science and Medicine, 51,* 1543–1554.

Smail, D. (1996). *How to survive without psychotherapy.* London: Constable.

Smail, D. (2005). *Power, interest and psychology: Elements of a social materialist understanding of distress.* Ross-on-Wye: PCCS Books.

Snape, M. C. (1997). Reactions to a traumatic event: The good, the bad and the ugly? *Psychology, Health and Medicine, 2,* 237–242.

Snyder, C. R. (Ed.) (2000). *Handbook of hope: Theory, measures, and applications.* San Diego, CA: Academic Press.

Snyder, C. R., & Lopez, S. J. (Eds.) (2002). *Handbook of positive psychology.* New York: Oxford University Press.

Snyder, C. R., & Lopez, S. J. (in press). *Positive psychology.* Thousand Oaks, CA: Sage.

Sternberg, R. J. (1998). A balance theory of wisdom. *Review of General Psychology, 2,* 347–365.

Sternberg, R. J., & Grigorenko, E. L. (2001). Unified psychology. *American Psychologist, 56,* 1069–1079.

Stewart, I. (1989). *Transactional analysis counselling in action.* London: Sage.

Taylor, E. (2001). Positive psychology and humanistic psychology: A reply to Seligman. *Journal of Humanistic Psychology, 41,* 13–29.

Taylor, S. E. (1983). Adjustment to threatening events: A theory of cognitive adaptation. *American Psychologist, 38,* 1161–1173.

Taylor, S. E., & Sherman, D. K. (2004). Positive psychology and health psychology: A fruitful liaison. In P. A. Linley, & S. Joseph (Eds.), *Positive psychology in practice* (pp. 305–319). Hoboken, NJ: John Wiley & Sons.

Taylor, S. E., Lichtman, R. R., & Wood, J. V. (1984). Attributions, beliefs about control, and adjustment to breast cancer. *Journal of Personality and Social Psychology, 46,* 489–502.

Taylor, S. E., Kemeny, M. E., Reed, G. M., & Aspinwall, L. G. (1991). Assault on the self: Positive illusions and adjustment to threatening events. In J. Strauss, & G. R. Goethals (Eds.), *The self: Interdisciplinary approaches* (pp. 239–254). New York: Springer-Verlag.

Teasdale, J. D., Segal, Z. V., Williams, J. M. G., Ridgeway, V. A., Soulsby, J. M., & Lau, M. A. (2000). Prevention of relapse/recurrence in major depression by mindfulness-based cognitive therapy. *Journal of Consulting and Clinical Psychology, 68,* 615–623.

Teasdale, J. D., Moore, R. G., Hayhurst, H., Pope, M., Williams, S., & Segal, Z. V. (2002). Metacognitive awareness and prevention of relapse in depression: Empirical evidence. *Journal of Consulting and Clinical Psychology, 70,* 275–287.

Tedeschi, R. G., & Calhoun, L. G. (1995). *Trauma and transformation: Growing in the aftermath of suffering.* Thousand Oaks, CA: Sage.

Tedeschi, R. G., & Calhoun, L. G. (1996). The posttraumatic growth inventory: Measuring the positive legacy of trauma. *Journal of Traumatic Stress, 9,* 455–471.

Tedeschi, R. G., & Calhoun, L. G. (2004). A clinical approach to post-traumatic growth. In P. A. Linley, & S. Joseph (Eds.), *Positive psychology in practice* (pp. 405–419). Hoboken, NJ: John Wiley & Sons.

Tedeschi, R. G., Park, C. L., & Calhoun, L. G. (Eds.) (1998a). *Post-traumatic growth: Positive changes in the aftermath of crisis.* Mahwah, NJ: Lawrence Erlbaum.

Tedeschi, R. G., Park, C. L., & Calhoun, L. G. (1998b). *Posttraumatic growth: Conceptual issues.* In R. G. Tedeschi, C. L. Park, & L. G. Calhoun (Eds.), *Posttraumatic growth: Positive changes in the aftermath of crisis.* Mahwah, NJ: Lawrence Erlbaum.

Tennen, H., Affleck, G., Urrows, S., Higgins, P., & Mendola, R. (1992). Perceiving control, construing benefits, and daily processes in rheumatoid arthritis. *Canadian Journal of Behavioral Science, 24,* 186–203.

Thompson, M. (2000). Life after rape: A chance to speak? *Sexual and Relationship Therapy, 15,* 325–343.

Thorne, B. (1992). *Carl Rogers.* London: Sage.

Thorne, B., & Lambers, E. (Eds.) (1998). *Person-centred therapy: A European perspective*. London: Sage.

Totton, N. (2004). Two ways of being helpful. *Counselling and Psychotherapy Journal, 15*, 5–9.

Truax, C. B., & Mitchell, K. M. (1971). Research on certain therapist interpersonal skills in relation to process and outcome. In A. E. Bergin, and S. L. Garfield (Eds.), *Handbook of psychotherapy and behavior change* (pp. 299–344). New York: John Wiley & Sons.

Updegraff, J. A., Taylor, S. E., Kemeny, M. E., & Wyatt, G. E. (2002). Positive and negative effects of HIV infection in women with low socioeconomic resources. *Personality and Social Psychology Bulletin, 28*, 382–394.

Van Werde, D. (1998). 'Anchorage' as a core concept in working with psychotic people. In B. Thorne, & E. Lambers (Eds.), *Person-centred therapy: A European perspective*. London: Sage.

Van Werde, D. (2005). Facing psychotic functioning: Person-centred contact work in residential psychiatric care. In S. Joseph, & R. Worsley (Eds.), *Person-centred psychopathology: A positive psychology of mental health* (pp. 158–168). Ross-on-Wye: PCCS Books.

Veenhoven, R. (2004). Happiness as a public policy aim: The greatest happiness principle. In P. A. Linley, & S. Joseph (Eds.), *Positive psychology in practice* (pp. 658–678). Hoboken, NJ: John Wiley & Sons.

Wampold, B. E. (2001). *The great psychotherapy debate: Models, methods, and findings*. Mahwah, NJ: Lawrence Erlbaum.

Ward, T., & Mann, R. (2004). Good lives and the rehabilitation of offenders: A positive approach to sex offender treatment. In P. A. Linley, & S. Joseph (Eds.), *Positive psychology in practice* (pp. 598–616). Hoboken, NJ: John Wiley & Sons.

Warner, M. (2005). A person-centred view of human nature, wellness, and psychopathology. In S. Joseph, & R. Worsley (Eds.), *Person-centred psychopathology: A positive psychology of mental health* (pp. 91–109). Ross-on-Wye: PCCS Books.

Waterman, A. S. (1993). Two conceptions of happiness: Contrasts of personal expressiveness (eudaemonia) and hedonic enjoyment. *Journal of Personality and Social Psychology, 64*, 678–691.

Weiss, T. (2002). Posttraumatic growth in women with breast cancer and their husbands: An intersubjective validation study. *Journal of Psychosocial Oncology, 20*, 65–80.

White, R. W. (1959). Motivation reconsidered: The concept of competence. *Psychological Review, 66*, 297–333.

Wilkins, P. (2005a). Person-centred theory and 'mental illness'. In S. Joseph, & R. Worsley (Eds.), *Person-centred psychopathology: A positive psychology of mental health* (pp. 43–59). Ross-on-Wye: PCCS Books.

Wilkins, P. (2005b). Assessment and 'diagnosis' in person-centred therapy. In S. Joseph, & R. Worsley (Eds.), *Person-centred psychopathology: A positive psychology of mental health* (pp. 128–145). Ross-on-Wye: PCCS Books.

Williams, G. C., Cox, E. M., Heberg, V. A., & Deci, E. L. (2000). Extrinsic life goals and health-risk behaviors among adolescents. *Journal of Applied Social Psychology, 30,* 1756–1771.

Woodward, C., & Joseph, S. (2003). Positive change processes and posttraumatic growth in people who have experienced childhood abuse: Understanding vehicles of change. *Psychology and Psychotherapy: Theory, Research and Practice, 76,* 267–283.

Worsley, R. (2001). *Process work in person-centred therapy.* Basingstoke: Palgrave.

Worsley, R. (2004). Integrating with integrity. In P. Sanders (2004). *The tribes of the person-centred nation: An introduction to the schools of therapy related to the person-centred approach* (pp. 125–148). Ross-on-Wye: PCCS Books.

Worsley, R. (2005). The concept of evil as a key to the therapists use of self. In S. Joseph, & R. Worsley (Eds.), *Person-centred psychopathology: A positive psychology of mental health* (pp. 146–157). Ross-on-Wye: PCCS Books.

Wyatt, G. (Ed.), (2001). *Rogers' therapeutic conditions: Evolution, theory and practice. Volume 1: Congruence.* Ross-on-Wye: PCCS Books.

Wyatt, G., & Sanders, P. (Eds.) (2001). *Rogers' therapeutic conditions: Evolution, theory and practice. Volume 4: Contact and perception.* Ross-on-Wye: PCCS Books.

Yalom, I. (1980). *Existential therapy.* New York: Basic Books.

Yalom, I. (1989). *Love's executioner and other tales of psychotherapy.* London: Penguin.

Yalom, I. D. (2001). *The gift of therapy: Reflections on being a therapist.* London: Piatkus.

Yalom, I. D., & Lieberman, M. A. (1991). Bereavement and heightened existential awareness. *Psychiatry, 54,* 334–345.

Zeig, J. K. (1987). *The evolution of psychotherapy.* New York: Brunner/Mazel.

Zenmore, R., Rinholm, J., Shepel, L. F., & Richards, M. (1989). Some social and emotional consequences of breast cancer and mastectomy: A content analysis of 87 interviews. *Journal of Psychosocial Oncology, 7,* 33–45.

Author index

Subject index

Note: page numbers in *italics* refer to information contained in tables and boxes.